The World Health Organization is a specialized agency of the United Nations with primary responsibility for international health matters and public health. Through this organization, which was created in 1948, the health professions of some 170 countries exchange their knowledge and experience with the aim of making possible the attainment by all citizens of the world by the year 2000 of a level of health that will permit them to lead a socially and economically productive life.

By means of direct technical cooperation with its Member States, and by stimulating such cooperation among them, WHO promotes the development of comprehensive health services, the prevention and control of diseases, the improvement of environmental conditions, the development of human resources for health, the coordination and development of biomedical and health services research, and the planning and implementation of health programmes.

These broad fields of endeavour encompass a wide variety of activities, such as developing systems of primary health care that reach the whole population of Member countries; promoting the health of mothers and children; combating malnutrition; controlling malaria and other communicable diseases including tuberculosis and leprosy; coordinating the global strategy for the prevention and control of AIDS; having achieved the eradication of smallpox, promoting mass immunization against a number of other preventable diseases; improving mental health; providing safe water supplies; and training health personnel of all categories.

Progress towards better health throughout the world also demands international cooperation in such matters as establishing international standards for biological substances, pesticides and pharmaceuticals; formulating environmental health criteria; recommending international non-proprietary names for drugs; administering the International Health Regulations; revising the International Statistical Classification of Diseases and Related Health Problems; and collecting and disseminating health statistical information.

Reflecting the concerns and priorities of the Organization and its Member States, WHO publications provide authoritative information and guidance aimed at promoting and protecting health and preventing and controlling disease.

# A guide to the development of on-site sanitation

R. Franceys, J. Pickford & R. Reed

*Water, Engineering and Development Centre*
*Loughborough University of Technology*
*Loughborough, England*

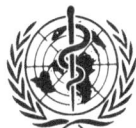

World Health Organization
Geneva
1992

WHO Library Cataloguing in Publication Data

Franceys, R.
  A guide to the development of on-site sanitation / R. Franceys,
J. Pickford & R. Reed

  1.Sanitation   2.Toilet facilities   3.Waste disposal, Fluid —
methods  I.Pickford, J.  II.Reed, R.  III.Title

  ISBN 92 4 154443 0     (NLM Classification: WA 778)

TYPESET IN INDIA
PRINTED IN ENGLAND
91/8829—Macmillan/Clays—7000

# Contents

**Part II. Detailed design, construction, operation and maintenance**

# Preface

For nearly thirty years, the names Wagner and Lanoix have recurred time and time again in connection with water supply and excreta disposal for rural areas and small communities. Their two volumes published by the World Health Organization in the late 1950s (Wagner & Lanoix, 1958, 1959) have stood the test of time.

Since their publication, there has been a massive increase in interest in water supply and sanitation, partly associated with the International Drinking Water Supply and Sanitation Decade (1981–1990). Many countries prepared programmes for the Decade that included optimistic forecasts for the provision of sanitation, but achieving the objectives has proved to be difficult. The majority of people living in rural areas and on the urban fringes in developing countries still lack satisfactory sanitation.

Some excellent publications, dealing with various aspects of appropriate technology for sanitation, have been produced by the World Bank and others. Much of the technology is a refinement of already known and practised methods, based on experience in a number of developing countries in Africa, Asia and Latin America. However, emphasis has been given to socioeconomic aspects of planning and implementing sanitation improvements.

This publication has therefore been prepared in response to these developments, as an update of Wagner & Lanoix's work, on which it draws heavily. The change of title is intended to focus attention on sanitation facilities on the householder's property, which are appropriate for some urban areas, as well as rural areas and small communities.

The book has three parts. Part I deals with the background to sanitation—health, sociological, financial and institutional issues, and the technologies available for excreta disposal. Part II provides in-depth technical information about the design, construction, operation and maintenance of the major types of on-site sanitation facility, while Part III describes the planning and development processes involved in projects and programmes. Annexes on reuse of excreta and sullage disposal are also included; although connected with on-site sanitation, these are primarily off-site activities.

The book has been compiled with the needs of many different readers in mind. The authors hope that it will prove useful for engineers, medical officers and sanitarians in the field, and also for administrators, health personnel, planners, architects, and many others who are concerned with improving sanitation in rural areas and underprivileged urban communities in developing countries.

The views expressed in this publication reflect the authors' field experience in many developing countries, supplemented by discussion with other workers and study of recent publications. The book in its final form has greatly benefited from the comments of the reviewers listed in Annex 3, whose experience and knowledge are internationally recognized. Special thanks are due to Mr J. N. Lanoix for his thorough review and comments, and to M. Bell, A. Coad, A. Cotton, M. Ince and M. Smith of WEDC for their invaluable input.

Although every effort has been made to represent a world view, the authors have been constantly aware of great variations in practices in different continents, countries and districts. Sometimes what is quite satisfactory for one community is rejected by other people living nearby. When applying the information given in this book it is wise to follow the advice of Dr E. F. Schumacher: "Find out what the people are doing, and help them to do it better."

# PART I
# Foundations of sanitary practice

CHAPTER 1
# The need for on-site sanitation

## Introduction

"Sanitation" refers to all conditions that affect health, especially with regard to dirt and infection and specifically to the drainage and disposal of sewage and refuse from houses (*The Concise Oxford Dictionary*). At its first meeting in 1950, the WHO Expert Committee on Environmental Sanitation defined environmental sanitation as including the control of community water supplies, excreta and wastewater disposal, refuse disposal, vectors of disease, housing conditions, food supplies and handling, atmospheric conditions, and the safety of the working environment. Environmental problems have since grown in complexity, especially with the advent of radiation and chemical hazards. Meanwhile, the world's needs for basic sanitation services (i.e., drinking-water supply, excreta and wastewater disposal) have greatly increased as a result of rapid population growth and higher expectations. This led to the designation by the United Nations of the International Drinking Water Supply and Sanitation Decade (1981–1990).

There has been considerable awareness of community water supply needs, but the problems of excreta and wastewater disposal have received less attention. In order to focus attention on these problems, "sanitation" became used and understood by people worldwide to refer only to excreta and wastewater disposal. A WHO Study Group in 1986 formally adopted this meaning by defining sanitation as "the means of collecting and disposing of excreta and community liquid wastes in a hygienic way so as not to endanger the health of individuals and the community as a whole" (WHO, 1987a). Hygienic disposal that does not endanger health should be the underlying objective of all sanitation programmes.

The cost of a sewerage system (which is usually more than four times that of on-site alternatives) and its requirement of a piped water supply preclude its adoption in the many communities in developing countries that lack adequate sanitation. On-site disposal, dealing with excreta where it is deposited, can provide a hygienic and satisfactory solution for such communities.

Safe disposal of excreta is of paramount importance for health and welfare and also for the social and environmental effects it may have in the communities involved. Its provision was listed by the WHO Expert Committee on Environmental Sanitation in 1954 among the first basic steps that should be taken towards ensuring a safe environment (WHO, 1954). More recently a WHO Expert Committee on the

Prevention and Control of Parasitic Infections (WHO, 1987b) stressed that "the provision of sanitary facilities for excreta disposal and their proper use are necessary components of any programme aimed at controlling intestinal parasites. In many areas, sanitation is the most urgent health need and those concerned with the control of intestinal parasitic infections are urged to promote intersectoral collaboration between health care authorities and those responsible for the provision of sanitation facilities and water supply at the community level."

## Historical evidence

There is historical evidence from the industrialized world of the need for sanitation as a high priority for health protection. For example, in England in the nineteenth century, exposure to water-related infections was reduced when government-sponsored environmental measures were taken following enactment of public health legislation.

## The present situation

Improved sanitation and domestic water supply warrant high priority for investment in developing countries where they are at the forefront of health improvements in both rural and urban communities. The importance attached to sanitation is part of a movement towards satisfaction of basic human needs—health care, housing, clean water, appropriate sanitation and adequate food. This movement has been instrumental in promoting a shift from curative to preventive medicine and in the designation of the 1980s as the International Drinking Water Supply and Sanitation Decade.

### Decade approaches

The decision to designate the Decade was taken at the United Nations Water Conference held in Mar del Plata in 1977. The Conference also agreed a plan of action, recommending that national programmes should give priority to:

- the rural and urban underserved populations;
- application of self-reliant and self-sustaining programmes;
- use of socially relevant systems;
- association of the community in all stages of development;
- complementarity of sanitation with water supply; and
- the association of water supply and sanitation with health and other sector programmes.

### The shortfall in sanitation

The percentage of the total population in the developing countries of the WHO Regions who do not have adequate sanitation is shown in

4

**Table 1.1. Percentage of the population without adequate sanitation**[a]

| WHO region | 1970 Urban | 1970 Rural | 1975 Urban | 1975 Rural | 1980 Urban | 1980 Rural | 1988 Urban | 1988 Rural |
|---|---|---|---|---|---|---|---|---|
| Africa | 53 | 77 | 25 | 72 | 46 | 80 | 46 | 79 |
| Americas | 24 | 76 | 20 | 75 | 44 | 80 | 10 | 69 |
| Eastern Mediterranean | 38 | 88 | 37 | 86 | 43 | 93 | 6 | 80 |
| South-East Asia | 67 | 96 | 69 | 96 | 70 | 94 | 59 | 89 |
| Western Pacific | 19 | 81 | 19 | 57 | 7 | 37 | 11 | 31 |
| Global total | 46 | 91 | 50 | 89 | 50 | 87 | 33 | 81 |

[a] From WHO, 1990.

Table 1.1, which is derived from statistics available to the Organization (WHO, 1990).

Notwithstanding some inaccuracies in reporting, there is abundant evidence that the scale of the problem is greatest in countries with a low gross national product (GNP) and especially in rural communities. There are also marked disparities in environmental conditions and in standards of health within the developing countries and particularly in the major cities.

## Problems of urban growth

Rates of urban growth of greater than 5% per year have produced concentrations of poor people in city-centre slums and in squatter areas on the periphery of towns and cities. Health risks are high in these areas. High-density living promotes the spread of airborne respiratory infections and hygiene-related diseases such as diarrhoea. Malnutrition is common and hence people are more susceptible to water-related infections. Such infections can spread rapidly since water sources are liable to faecal pollution. A major challenge for those concerned with environmental health is the design and introduction of excreta disposal systems appropriate to these high-density, low-income communities.

## Rural problems

There is an equal need for the hygienic disposal of excreta and the promotion of health in rural areas. Rural communities may have evolved what they perceive to be satisfactory disposal systems, but the introduction of improved sanitation facilities can form a useful part of broader rural development programmes. The level of sanitation provision should be linked to that of other facilities in the community, and to the community's ability to support (financially and culturally) and maintain such provisions.

## Constraints

The many constraints on improving health through better sanitation centre on the political, economic, social and cultural contexts of health and disease. Worldwide surveys conducted by WHO identified the following as the most serious constraints:

— funding limitations;
— insufficiency of trained personnel;
— operation and maintenance;
— logistics;
— inadequate cost-recovery framework;
— insufficient health education efforts;
— inappropriate institutional framework;
— intermittent water service;
— non-involvement of communities.

## Priorities

There are four main targets for sanitation programmes: rural development, urban upgrading, periurban shanty and squatter upgrading, and new urban development. Programmes for these areas may be similar in content or approach. For example, both rural and shanty town development may have a high level of community contribution in labour, yet they may be very different in the input of health education, introduction or enhancing awareness of new technologies, development of managerial structure, and provision of finance.

Questions have arisen concerning the kinds of technology that are most appropriate to the communities to be served and how this technology can best be introduced. The need for technical specialists to be aware of the social and cultural context of engineering interventions has been emphasized together with the need for popular participation in project design and implementation. Concepts such as grass-roots development, based on an approach that builds from below, have offered a challenge to the top-down approach based on decisions made at high managerial levels. The former is critical in sanitation programmes, since the effectiveness of these programmes depends not merely on community support but, more particularly, on the consent and commitment of households and individual users. Further, in sanitation programmes, technical and social decisions are closely interrelated.

# CHAPTER 2

# Sanitation and disease transmission

## Diseases associated with excreta and wastewater

### Sources of disease

The inadequate and insanitary disposal of infected human faeces leads to the contamination of the ground and of sources of water. Often it provides the sites and the opportunity for certain species of flies and mosquitos to lay their eggs, to breed, or to feed on the exposed material and to carry infection. It also attracts domestic animals, rodents and other vermin which spread the faeces and with them the potential for disease. In addition it sometimes creates intolerable nuisances of both odour and sight.

There are a number of diseases related to excreta and wastewater which commonly affect people in the developing countries and which can be subdivided into communicable and noncommunicable diseases.

### Communicable diseases

The major communicable diseases whose incidence can be reduced by the introduction of safe excreta disposal are intestinal infections and helminth infestations, including cholera, typhoid and paratyphoid fevers, dysentery and diarrhoea, hookworm, schistosomiasis and filariasis.

Table 2.1 lists some of the pathogenic organisms frequently found in faeces, urine and sullage (greywater).

#### High-risk groups

Those most at risk of these diseases are children under five years of age, as their immune systems are not fully developed and may be further impaired by malnutrition. The diarrhoeal diseases are by far the major underlying cause of mortality in this age group, accounting for some 4 million deaths each year.

In 1973, children in Brazil under one year of age totalled less than one-fifth of the population but suffered almost four-fifths of all deaths, while in the United States of America this age group represented 8.8% of the population and suffered only 4.3% of deaths (Berg, 1973).

There is no doubt that improving the sanitation within a community should lead to an improvement in health, but it is difficult

**Table 2.1. Occurrence of some pathogens in urine,[a] faeces and sullage[b]**

| Pathogen | Common name for infection caused | Present in: | | |
|---|---|---|---|---|
| | | urine | faeces | sullage |
| Bacteria | | | | |
| Escherichia coli | diarrhoea | * | * | * |
| Leptospira interrogans | leptospirosis | * | | |
| Salmonella typhi | typhoid | * | * | * |
| Shigella spp | shigellosis | | * | |
| Vibrio cholerae | cholera | | * | |
| Viruses | | | | |
| Poliovirus | poliomyelitis | | * | * |
| Rotaviruses | enteritis | | * | |
| Protozoa—amoeba or cysts | | | | |
| Entamoeba histolytica | amoebiasis | | * | * |
| Giardia intestinalis | giardiasis | | * | * |
| Helminths—parasite eggs | | | | |
| Ascaris lumbricoides | roundworm | | * | * |
| Fasciola hepatica | liver fluke | | * | |
| Ancylostoma duodenale | hookworm | | * | * |
| Necator americanus | hookworm | | * | * |
| Schistosoma spp | schistosomiasis | * | * | * |
| Taenia spp | tapeworm | | * | * |
| Trichuris trichiura | whipworm | | * | * |

[a] Urine is usually sterile; the presence of pathogens indicates either faecal pollution or host infection, principally with Salmonella typhi, Schistosoma haematobium or Leptospira.
[b] From Cheesebrough (1984), Sridhar et al. (1981) and Feachem et al. (1983).

to ascertain whether the impact would be direct or indirect. Often, provision of better sanitation is part of broader development activities within the community and, even if dissociated from improvement of the water supply, there are usually other factors that influence health which are introduced with sanitation changes, e.g., health and hygiene education (Blum & Feachem, 1983). The effect of these factors, such as increased handwashing or changes in attitudes to children's excreta, may be difficult to monitor and/or evaluate.

Table 2.2 gives details for different countries of infant and child deaths (including deaths from diarrhoea), life expectancy at birth, and the levels of poverty in both urban and rural areas. In general, these data reflect an interactive relationship between poverty/malnutrition and children's health. In turn, this relationship may be related to the level of sanitation in the children's environment. For instance, the incidence of diarrhoeal disease in children is affected by poor personal hygiene and environmental sanitation, and also by reduced resistance to disease in malnutrition. Diarrhoea leads to loss of weight, which is normally transitory in the well nourished but more persistent in the malnourished. Repeated infections can lead to increased malnutrition

**Table 2.2. Health indicators**[a]

| Country | Infant mortality rate per 1000 live births | | Child mortality per 1000 (1–5 years) | Life expectancy at birth (years) | | Population below poverty line (%) | |
|---|---|---|---|---|---|---|---|
| | 1983 | 1985 | | 1983 | 1985 | Urban | Rural |
| Bangladesh | 130 | 121 | 205 | 48 | 54 | 86 | 86 |
| Ecuador | 70 | 45 | 95 | 63 | 64 | 30 | 65 |
| Finland | 6 | 6 | 8 | 73 | 75 | — | — |
| Haiti | 130 | 125 | 190 | 53 | 54 | 55 | 78 |
| India | 110 | 114 | 165 | 53 | 54 | 40 | 51 |
| Malaysia | 30 | 17 | 41 | 67 | 70 | 13 | 38 |
| Nepal | 140 | 140 | 215 | 46 | 52 | 55 | 61 |
| Papua New Guinea | 75 | 72 | 105 | 53 | 50 | 10 | 75 |
| Paraguay | 45 | 30 | 65 | 65 | 65 | 19 | 50 |
| Philippines | 50 | 57 | 85 | 65 | 63 | 32 | 41 |
| Sierra Leone | 180 | 225 | 310 | 34 | 47 | — | 65 |
| Thailand | 48 | 12 | 60 | 63 | 63 | 15 | 34 |
| Trinidad and Tobago | 24 | 19 | 28 | 70 | 67 | — | 39 |
| United Kingdom | 10 | 12 | 12 | 74 | 73 | — | — |

[a] From UNICEF (1986); WHO (1987c).

which in turn increases susceptibility to further infection; this may be referred to as the diarrhoea–malnutrition cycle.

## Noncommunicable diseases

In addition to pathogen content, the chemical composition of waste-water has to be considered because of its effects on crop growth and/or consumers. The number of components to be monitored (e.g., heavy metals, organic compounds, detergents, etc.) is greater in industrialized urban areas than in rural areas. Nitrate content is important, however, in all areas because of the possible effects of its accumulation, in both surface and groundwater, on human health (methaemoglobin-aemia in infants), and on the ecological balance in waters receiving run-off or effluent high in nitrates. Although the major human activity resulting in the increase of nitrate levels is the use of chemical fertilizers, poor sanitation or misuse of wastewater can contribute to or, in exceptional cases, be the major determinant of nitrate levels, particularly in groundwater.

## How disease is carried from excreta

### Transmission of diseases

Humans themselves are the main reservoir of most diseases that affect them. Transmission of excreta-related diseases from one host to

**Fig. 2.1. Transmission routes for pathogens found in excreta**

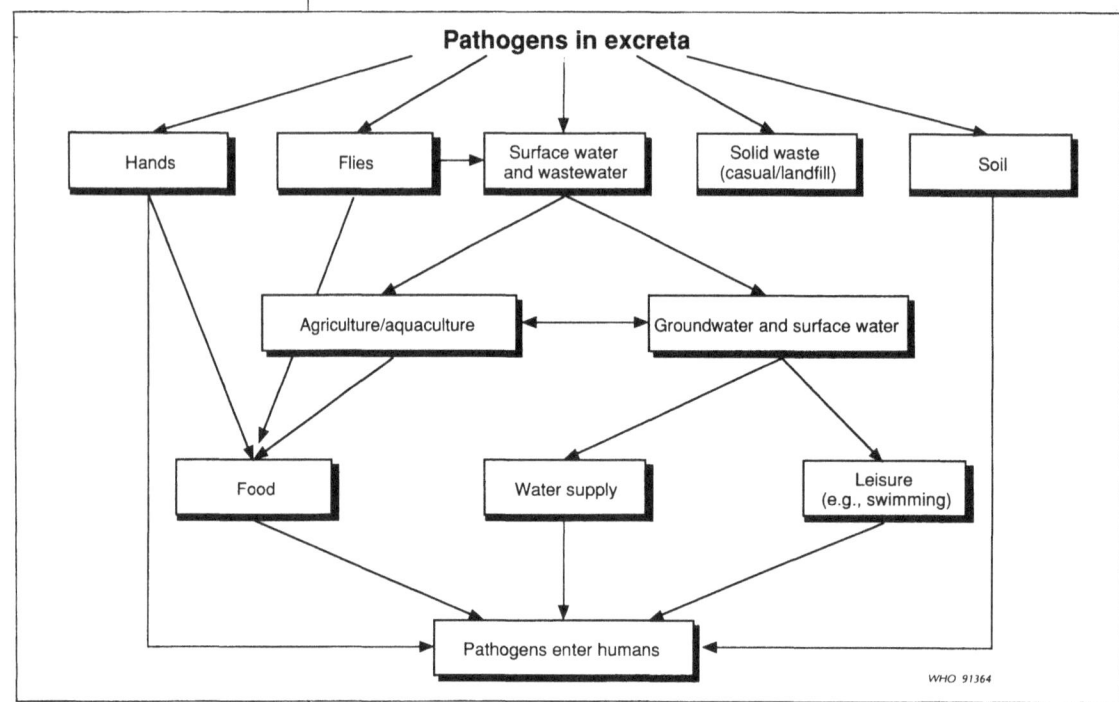

**Table 2.3. Morbidity and mortality associated with various excreta-related diseases**

| Disease | Morbidity | Mortality (no. of deaths per year) | Population at risk |
|---|---|---|---|
| **Waterborne and water-washed** | | | |
| diarrhoea | 1500 million or more episodes in children under 5 years | 4 million in children under 5 years | More than 2000 million |
| poliomyelitis | 204 000 | 25 000 | |
| enteric fevers (typhoid, paratyphoid) | 500 000–1 million | 25 000 | |
| roundworm | 800–1000 million infections | 20 000 | |
| **Water-based** | | | |
| schistosomiasis | 200 million | More than 200 000 | 500–600 million |
| **Soil-based** | | | |
| hookworm | 900 million infections | 50 000 | |

another (or the same host) normally follows one of the routes shown in Fig. 2.1. Poor domestic and personal hygiene, indicated by routes involving food and hands, often diminishes or even negates any positive impact of improved excreta disposal on community health. As shown in the figure, most routes for transmission of excreta-related diseases are the same as those for water-related diseases, being dependent on faecal–oral transmission (waterborne and water-washed) and skin penetration (water-based with an aquatic host; soil-based but not faecal–oral; and insect vector with vector breeding on excreta or in dirty water). Table 2.3 gives examples of excreta-related diseases and data on the number of infections and deaths per year.

As Table 2.3 illustrates, diarrhoeal diseases and helminth infections account for the greatest number of cases per year although there is a considerable difference in the levels of debility they produce. Schistosomiasis has relatively high rates of infection and death. The socioeconomic impact of these diseases should not be ignored or underestimated. To illustrate this further, schistosomiasis will be considered in greater detail.

### Schistosomiasis

Schistosomiasis is acquired through repeated contact with surface water contaminated with human excreta (both urine and faeces) containing schistosomes (WHO, 1985). Contact can be via agriculture, aquaculture, leisure activities (particularly swimming), collection of water, washing and bathing. Of the parasitic diseases, schistosomiasis ranks second in terms of socioeconomic and public health importance in tropical and subtropical areas, immediately behind malaria.

In 1990, schistosomiasis was reported to be endemic in 76 developing countries. Over 200 million people in rural and agricultural areas were estimated to be infected, while 500–600 million more were at risk of becoming infected, because of poverty, ignorance, substandard hygiene, and poor housing with few, if any, sanitary facilities.

People with light infections as well as those with obvious symptoms suffer weakness and lethargy, which decrease their capacity for work and productivity.

As shown in Fig. 2.2, the parasite develops in snails, the intermediate hosts. The free-swimming stage of the parasite penetrates the skin of humans and, if infection is heavy, the disease develops. The incidence of diseases such as schistosomiasis should be much reduced by the provision of sanitation. However, for this disease, as for many others, additional measures including the provision of safe drinking-water can also interrupt transmission by reducing contact with infested water. People living in endemic areas can benefit greatly from health education aimed at increasing their understanding of their role in transmission, and the importance of the use of latrines. Since young children are often most heavily infected, early use of latrines, especially in schools, will promote healthy habits.

**Fig. 2.2. The cycle of transmission of schistosomiasis**

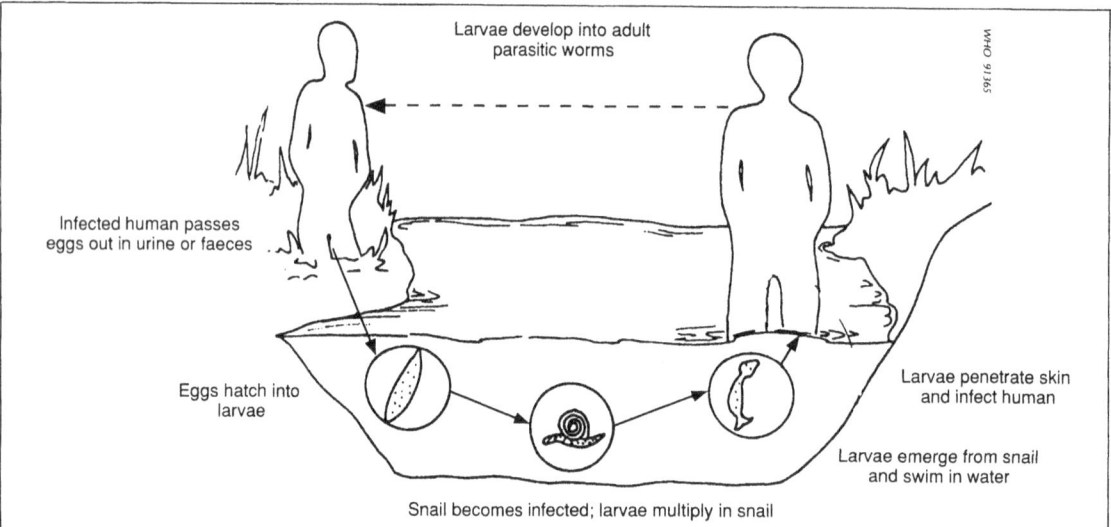

## Reuse of excreta and wastewater in agriculture

Sanitation is not always the only factor to be considered when relating excreta disposal to disease transmission within and between communities. The reuse of excreta (untreated or treated to differing extents) as a fertilizer, and reuse of wastewater (including sullage water) for many purposes, but especially for irrigation, may also contribute to the incidence of excreta-related diseases. In many countries where the demand for water is greater than the supply, use of wastewater for irrigation of crops for consumption by animals or humans can have a major impact on community health. This is especially important in areas with poor soils and insufficient income for purchase of commercial fertilizers and conditioners, where the use of human as well as animal excreta to condition and fertilize soil is actively encouraged. With such practices the degree of the hazard is dependent on several parameters including:

— the level (or lack) of treatment prior to reuse;
— the nature of the crop;
— the method of irrigation;
— the extent of reuse;
— the incidence and type of disease in the area;
— air, soil and water conditions.

The groups most at risk of infection will also depend on these factors and on other agricultural practices. The diseases that may show the greatest increase in incidence where reuse is practised are helminth infestations, particularly hookworm, roundworm and whip-worm; schistosomiasis may also increase markedly in some circumstances. Bacterial infections, such as cholera and diarrhoea, are affected to a much smaller degree, with the incidence of viral infections being least affected by these practices (Mara & Cairncross, 1989; WHO, 1989).

## Epidemiological characteristics of pathogens

### Pathogen survival

The survival times and other epidemiological characteristics of organisms in different media are given in Table 2.4; it should be noted that these periods are approximate, being dependent on local factors such as the climate and the number (concentration) and species of organisms.

### Pathogen infectivity and latency

In addition to knowing how long the infectious agent may survive, i.e., its persistence, knowledge of the infectivity and latency of the organism is of value. Some pathogens remain infective for only short periods after being excreted, yet the incidence of associated disease is high. This may be attributable to the low infectious dose of the organism,

**Table 2.4. The epidemiological characteristics of excreted pathogens**[a]

| Pathogen | Latency period | $ID_{50}$[b] | Survival times for pathogens in· | | |
|---|---|---|---|---|---|
| | | | wastewater | soil | crops |
| Bacteria | 0 | $>10^4$ | | few days to 3 months | |
| *Vibrio cholerae* | 0 | $10^8$ | ~1 month | <3 weeks | <5 days |
| Faecal coliform | 0 | ~$10^9$ | ~3 months | <2 months | <1 month |
| Viruses | 0 | unknown | months | months | 1–2 months |
| Enteroviruses[c] | 0 | 100 | ~3 months | <3 months | <2 months |
| Protozoa (cysts) | 0 | 10–100 | | few days to few weeks | |
| *Entamoeba* spp | 0 | 10–100 | 25 days | <3 weeks | <10 days |
| Helminths[d] | variable | 1–100 | months | months | months |
| *Ancylostoma* spp | 1 week | 1 | 3 months | <3 months | <1 month |
| *Ascaris* spp | 10 days | several | ~1 year | many months | <3 months |
| Flukes[e] | 6–8 weeks | several | life of host[f] | hours[f] | hours[f] |

[a] Sources: Feachem et al. (1983); WHO (1987a).
[b] The $ID_{50}$ is the number of organisms required to cause the development of clinical symptoms in 50% of individuals.
[c] Including coxsackieviruses, echoviruses and polioviruses.
[d] Eggs or larvae/cercariae.
[e] Excluding *Fasciola hepatica* but including *Schistosoma* spp.
[f] Outside the aquatic host, the pathogen survives for only a few hours. In the host, survival is for the life of the host.

e.g., protozoal cysts. The latency of an organism (i.e., the period between leaving a host and becoming infective) can vary from zero for some bacterial infections to weeks for some helminth eggs. For example, schistosome eggs have a latency of a few weeks during which time they develop in an intermediate host into the infective, free-swimming cercariae (Fig. 2.2); however, both the eggs and the cercariae have a persistence of only a few hours if they do not enter a new host (intermediate or human). In contrast, *Ascaris* eggs can become infective within ten days of being excreted (latency) but may remain in the soil for at least a year and still be infective (persistence).

## Control of excreta-related diseases

If transmission is blocked at one or more points, excreta-related diseases can be controlled or possibly eradicated. Sanitation provides one such block. For example, water-seal slabs in latrines reduce the breeding sites for culicine mosquitos, vectors of filariasis; treatment of excreta prior to its disposal can kill the eggs and cysts of many human parasites (*Ascaris*, *Entamoeba*, and *Schistosoma* spp), thus preventing contamination of both ground and water.

## Relationship of health to disposal method

The technical objective of sanitary excreta disposal is to isolate faeces so that the infectious agents in them cannot reach a new host. The method chosen for any particular area or region will depend on many factors including the local geology and hydrogeology, the culture and preferences of the communities, the locally available raw materials and the cost (both short-term and long-term).

The types of disease that are endemic in an area should also be considered. The survival of endemic pathogens (eggs, cysts, infectious agents) and the destination or possible reuse of different products of disposal/treatment can have a great effect on incidence of disease in that area and, possibly, adjacent areas.

The possible sites for both negative and positive impacts on health, taking all the above parameters into consideration, should be considered during the planning stages of development projects to improve sanitation. This should ensure that the projects achieve the greatest possible effect on the incidence of diseases related to excreta and wastewater in the community.

CHAPTER 3
# Social and cultural considerations

The introduction of on-site sanitation systems is much more than the application of simple engineering techniques—it is an intervention that entails considerable social change. If sanitation improvements in rural and urban areas are to be widely accepted, the relevant social and cultural factors have to be taken into consideration during planning and implementation. It is therefore necessary to understand how a society functions, including the communities and households within it, and what factors promote change.

## Social structure

Consideration should be given to the institutions of a political, economic and social nature that are operating at the national and/or local level, such as government, the civil service, religious institutions, schools and colleges, and the family, and to the forms of leadership and authority that are generally accepted by the majority of the people. It is also important to consider the various roles and patterns of behaviour of individuals and social groups, and to determine who is traditionally responsible for such areas as water supplies, environmental hygiene, family health and children's defecation habits, etc.

## Cultural beliefs and practices

Group and community identity, gender roles, the relative importance attached to different forms of authority and the ways in which it is exercised are all influenced by culture, i.e., all that is passed down by human society including language, laws, customs, beliefs and moral standards. Culture shapes human behaviour in many different ways including the status attached to different roles and what is deemed to be acceptable personal and social behaviour. In many cultures, for example, the elderly command traditional authority and influence within the family and community.

As regards sanitation behaviour, defecation is often a private matter which people are unwilling to discuss openly, while the burying of faeces is widely practised to ward off evil spirits. Contact with faecal matter is unacceptable to certain individuals in societies where it is the responsibility of low-income or low-caste groups, while taboos may dictate that separate facilities should be provided for particular social groups.

A particular cultural practice to be considered, which has direct technical consequences, is the method of anal cleansing used by the community. Whether water, stones, corncobs or thick pieces of paper are used will affect the design of the sanitation system.

Culture also influences how people interpret and evaluate the environment in which they live. Investments in sanitation seek to improve health by providing a clean physical environment for households. There is a logical series of technical questions that need to be asked in order that acceptable technical solutions can be found. It may be confusing, therefore, when sanitation behaviour is found to vary widely between communities within the same physical environment. Predetermined rules cannot be applied. However, the sanitation behaviour of individuals usually has a rational basis, and people are often aware of the environmental causes of ill-health. Many societies have a detailed knowledge of the physical environment as a provider of resources for curative and preventive medicine and as a cause of illness. More than this, they have an understanding of the environment, not only in its physical sense, but also in relation to social and spiritual factors. This holistic view of the environment permeates many of the cultural beliefs and customs that impinge on both water use patterns and sanitation behaviour. Some illustrations of these beliefs are given below.

## Concepts of hygiene

Although communities may lack knowledge of modern medical explanations of disease, they often have concepts of what is pure and polluting. Of the water resources available to particular households for domestic purposes, running water may be most acceptable for drinking because it is exposed to the sunlight; it is considered to be "alive" and therefore "pure", while water in shallow wells, which does not have these attributes, is deemed suitable only for washing and cooking. Communities have been observed to use the environmental resources available to them, such as bamboo, to bring fast-flowing river water to their villages in preference to more convenient well water that is unacceptable in taste, colour and smell.

Concepts of clean and dirty, pure and polluting, are well developed in the major world religions, and have a ritual and spiritual significance as well as referring to a physical state. When people are told that new sanitation facilities will make their environment "cleaner", it is their own interpretation of this concept that will be used. "Clean" may have quite different meanings to project promoters and recipients. Thus "it is essential to look into traditional categories of cleanliness and dirtiness, purity and pollution before embarking on a campaign to motivate people to accept a project in improved . . . sanitation or to change their behaviour to comply with new standards of 'cleanliness'" (Simpson-Hebert, 1984).

## Beliefs about sanitation and disease

Evidence of the value attached by communities to cleanliness and, by implication, environmental sanitation is found in studies of diarrhoea. People's perceptions of its causes may be divided into three categories, physical, social and spiritual. In many cases, physical causes are identified and, although the germ theory is not explicitly stated, the faecal–oral transmission routes of diarrhoea appear to be understood. Households may associate diarrhoea with a polluted environment including uncovered food, dirty water and flies. Graphic descriptions of pollution have been quoted (de Zoysa et al., 1984):

— *"We have to drink the dam water where animals and children bathe and the dirty water makes us ill."*
— *"Flies sit on dirt which they eat then they come on to uncovered foods and spit on to foods which we eat."*

As on-site sanitation involves improving the physical environment, it may therefore be readily accepted as one means by which to reduce the incidence of disease.

Equally, social and spiritual causes are perceived to be important, and include, for example, female social indiscretions and witchcraft. But these three apparently unrelated causes of diarrhoea should not be interpreted as mutually exclusive or divergent approaches to disease. They are often closely interrelated in practice, within a holistic interpretation of the environment.

Efforts should be made to determine how a community's beliefs, knowledge, and control over the environment can be harnessed in a positive way. Careful judgement is required to distinguish between those beliefs and ritual behaviour that are conducive to good sanitation practice and those that need to be changed.

## Forces for change

All societies undergo adjustments in their social structure and culture over time. This may result from contact between societies or from alterations in the physical environment such as prolonged drought. Further, changes in development practice and in international aid influence national goals and priorities with respect to different sectors and regions. How change is brought about and what it is that changes are important issues that need to be addressed.

The profound impact of forces for change on diverse societies finds expression in patterns of apparently increasing uniformity between countries and cultures. In demographic terms, these include rapid rates of national population growth, and internal migration of people from rural to urban areas coupled with urban expansion.

## Responses to change

The responses of individuals and groups to urban life, to factory employment or to new technology are a product of the values, experiences and behaviour patterns that they have assimilated over time as members of particular communities and societies. Some groups and individuals are more open to change and more able to adapt to it than others. Decisions are taken to accept or resist an innovation on the basis of characteristics peculiar to the individual, household or group within the context of the local physical, social, economic, cultural and demographic environment.

Access to education may increase awareness of the health benefits of improved sanitation technology, while income will influence the ability of a household to acquire particular facilities. Personal experience and demonstration of alternative technologies may help to convince people that the benefits of the investment will outweigh any costs incurred. Community organizations and influential leaders can assist in marketing the concept by emphasizing factors valued locally. These may include the status attached to possessing a facility, or its functional value in terms of comfort. Equally, factors such as rapid increase in population which limits privacy may heighten the perceived need for innovations in sanitation.

People resist change for many reasons. There may be resentment towards outside "experts" who know little of local customs and who are perceived to benefit more from the innovation than local people. Leadership may not be united within a community. For example, those with traditional authority who fear a loss of power and status may oppose innovation strongly supported by political or educated elites. New technologies may be aesthetically unacceptable or conflict with established patterns of personal and social behaviour. Furthermore, households vary widely in the resources of money, labour and time available to them and have their own priorities. For those with limited resources, the costs in the short term of an apparently "low-cost" system may be too great when set against their need for food, shelter and clothing. In addition, in terms of capital investment latrines may be very costly for households if they take a long time to clean, are difficult to use or involve radical changes in social habits (Pacey, 1980). There may also be seasonal variations in the availability of money and labour. Thus the timing of the promotional aspects of a project in relation to, for example, agricultural seasons may be important in determining the local response.

The demographic composition, economic characteristics and attitudes to sanitation of individual households change over time. Experience shows that once people start to improve their houses their interest in latrines is likely to be aroused. Thus some households may be encouraged to install a latrine as one aspect of the modernization process. Projects should be flexible enough to allow households to invest in on-site sanitation not only when they feel motivated but also when they have the resources to do so. Indeed it may be most appropriate to introduce a range of on-site technologies within a particular community from which households can make a choice according to their own changing needs and priorities.

## Conclusion

To identify a demand for improved sanitation is more positive than to initiate a supply of technology that is deemed to be good for communities. The former depends upon cooperation between providers and beneficiaries which comes through dialogue and the exchange of information. Individual users are the ultimate decision-makers in the acceptance or rejection of new technology. It is they who determine the success of a project, since the value of the investment depends not only upon community support but, more particularly, on the consent of households and individual users. They need to be convinced that the benefits of improved sanitation, and the new technology with which it is associated, outweigh the costs. Equally, it is for providers to appreciate the social context and the constraints within which individual decisions are made. They must learn from communities about why improved sanitation may elicit negative responses and also the positive features of community values, beliefs and practices which can be harnessed to promote change.

CHAPTER 4
# Technical options

In this chapter various sanitation systems are introduced with a brief indication of their suitability for particular situations, the constraints on their use, and their disadvantages. The whole range of options is covered, including off-site systems and some that are not recommended because of the associated health risk and other disadvantages. Each community must choose the most feasible and convenient option to provide necessary health protection. Selecting the most appropriate option requires a thorough analysis of all factors including cost, cultural acceptability, simplicity of design and construction, operation and maintenance, and local availability of materials and skills. Further details of the design, construction, operation and maintenance of these systems are given in Part II.

## Open defecation

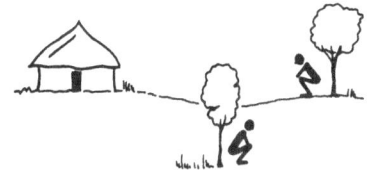

Where there are no latrines people resort to defecation in the open. This may be indiscriminate or in special places for defecation generally accepted by the community, such as defecation fields, rubbish and manure heaps, or under trees. Open defecation encourages flies, which spread faeces-related diseases. In moist ground the larvae of intestinal worms develop, and faeces and larvae may be carried by people and animals. Surface water run-off from places where people have defecated results in water pollution. In view of the health hazards created and the degradation of the environment, open defecation should not be tolerated in villages and other built-up areas. There are better options available that confine excreta in such a way that the cycle of reinfection from excreta-related diseases is broken.

## Shallow pit

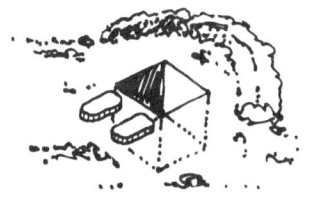

People working on farms may dig a small hole each time they defecate and then cover the faeces with soil. This is sometimes known as the "cat" method. Pits about 300 mm deep may be used for several weeks. Excavated soil is heaped beside the pit and some is put over the faeces after each use. Decomposition in shallow pits is rapid because of the large bacterial population in the topsoil, but flies breed in large numbers and hookworm larvae spread around the holes. Hookworm larvae can migrate upwards from excreta buried less than 1 m deep, to penetrate the soles of the feet of subsequent users.

| Advantages | Disadvantages |
|---|---|
| No cost | Considerable fly nuisance |
| Benefit to farmers as fertilizer | Spread of hookworm larvae |

## Simple pit latrine

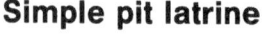

This consists of a slab over a pit which may be 2 m or more in depth. The slab should be firmly supported on all sides and raised above the surrounding ground so that surface water cannot enter the pit. If the sides of the pit are liable to collapse they should be lined. A squat hole in the slab or a seat is provided so that the excreta fall directly into the pit.

| Advantages | Disadvantages |
|---|---|
| Low cost | Considerable fly nuisance (and mosquito nuisance if the pit is wet) unless there is a tight-fitting cover over the squat hole when the latrine is not in use |
| Can be built by householder | |
| Needs no water for operation | |
| Easily understood | |
| | Smell |

## Borehole latrine

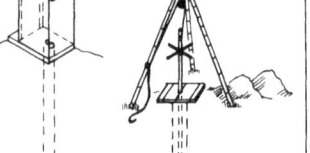

A borehole excavated by hand with an auger or by machine can be used as a latrine. The diameter is often about 400 mm and the depth 6–8 m.

| Advantages | Disadvantages |
|---|---|
| Can be excavated quickly if boring equipment is available | Sides liable to be fouled, with consequent fly nuisance |
| Suitable for short-term use, as in disaster situations | Short life owing to small cross-sectional area |
| | Greater risk of groundwater pollution owing to depth of hole |

## Ventilated pit latrine

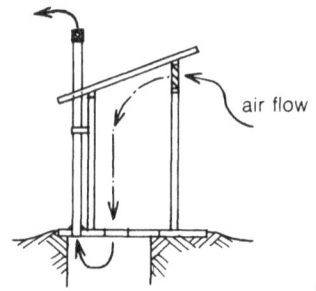
air flow

Fly and odour nuisance may be substantially reduced if the pit is ventilated by a pipe extending above the latrine roof, with fly-proof netting across the top. The inside of the superstructure is kept dark. Such latrines are known as ventilated improved pit (VIP) latrines.

| Advantages | Disadvantages |
|---|---|
| Low cost | Does not control mosquitos |
| Can be built by householder | Extra cost of providing vent pipe |
| Needs no water for operation | Need to keep interior dark |
| Easily understood | |
| Control of flies | |
| Absence of smell in latrines | |

## Pour-flush latrine

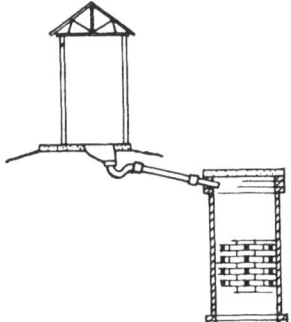

A latrine may be fitted with a trap providing a water seal, which is cleared of faeces by pouring in sufficient quantities of water to wash the solids into the pit and replenish the water seal. A water seal prevents flies, mosquitos and odours reaching the latrine from the pit. The pit may be offset from the latrine by providing a short length of pipe or covered channel from the pan to the pit. The pan of an offset pour-flush latrine is supported by the ground and the latrine may be within or attached to a house.

| Advantages | Disadvantages |
|---|---|
| Low cost | A reliable (even if limited) water supply must be available |
| Control of flies and mosquitos | |
| Absence of smell in latrine | Unsuitable where solid anal cleaning material is used |
| Contents of pit not visible | |
| Gives users the convenience of a WC | |
| Can be upgraded by connection to sewer when sewerage becomes available | |
| *Offset type* | |
| Pan supported by ground | |
| Latrine can be in house | |

## Single or double pit

In rural and low-density urban areas, the usual practice is to dig a second pit when the one in use is full to within half a metre of the slab. If the superstructure and slab are light and prefabricated they can be moved to a new pit. Otherwise a new superstructure and slab have to be constructed. The first pit is then filled up with soil. After two years, faeces in the first pit will have completely decomposed and even the

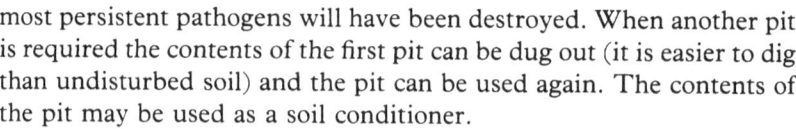

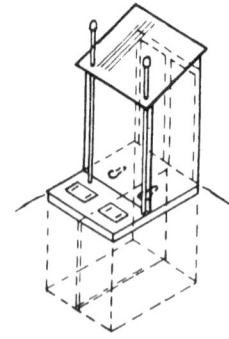

most persistent pathogens will have been destroyed. When another pit is required the contents of the first pit can be dug out (it is easier to dig than undisturbed soil) and the pit can be used again. The contents of the pit may be used as a soil conditioner.

Alternatively, two lined pits may be constructed, each large enough to take an accumulation of faecal solids over a period of two years or more. One pit is used until it is full, and then the second pit is used until that too is full, by which time the contents of the first pit can be removed and used as a fertilizer with no danger to health. The first pit can then be used again.

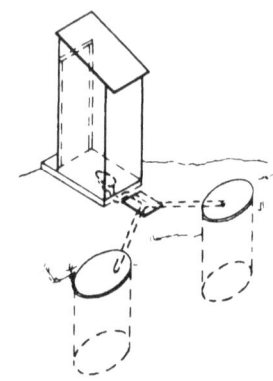

| Advantages of single pits | Advantages of double pits |
| --- | --- |
| Will last for several years if large enough | Once constructed the pits are more or less permanent |
| | Easy removal of solids from the pits as they are shallow |
| | Pit contents can be safely used as a soil conditioner after 2 years, without treatment |

## Composting latrine

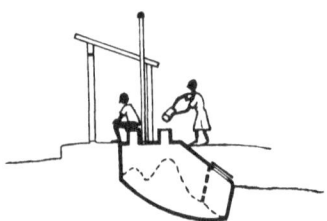

In this latrine, excreta fall into a watertight tank to which ash or vegetable matter is added. If the moisture content and chemical balance are controlled, the mixture will decompose to form a good soil conditioner in about four months. Pathogens are killed in the dry alkaline compost, which can be removed for application to the land as a fertilizer. There are two types of composting latrine: in one, compost is produced continuously, and in the other, two containers are used to produce it in batches.

| Advantages | Disadvantages |
| --- | --- |
| A valuable humus is produced | Careful operation is essential |
| | Urine has to be collected separately in the batch system |
| | Ash or vegetable matter must be added regularly |

## Septic tank

A septic tank is an underground watertight settling chamber into which raw sewage is delivered through a pipe from plumbing fixtures

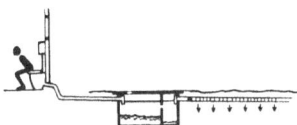

inside a house or other building. The sewage is partially treated in the tank by separation of solids to form sludge and scum. Effluent from the tank infiltrates into the ground through drains or a soakpit. The system works well where the soil is permeable and not liable to flooding or waterlogging, provided the sludge is removed at appropriate intervals to ensure that it does not occupy too great a proportion of the tank capacity.

| Advantages | Disadvantages |
|---|---|
| Gives the users the convenience of a WC | High cost |
| | Reliable and ample piped water required |
| | Only suitable for low-density housing |
| | Regular desludging required, and sludge needs careful handling |
| | Permeable soil required |

## Aqua-privy

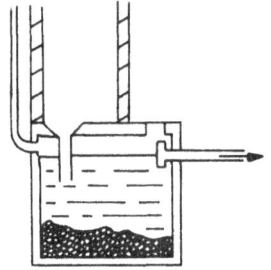

An aqua-privy has a watertight tank immediately under the latrine floor. Excreta drop directly into the tank through a pipe. The bottom of the pipe is submerged in the liquid in the tank, forming a water seal to prevent escape of flies, mosquitos and smell. The tank functions like a septic tank. Effluent usually infiltrates into the ground through a soakpit. Accumulated solids (sludge) must be removed regularly. Enough water must be added to compensate for evaporation and leakage losses.

| Advantages | Disadvantages |
|---|---|
| Does not need piped water on site | Water must be available nearby |
| Less expensive than a septic tank | More expensive than VIP or pour-flush latrine |
| | Fly, mosquito and smell nuisance if seal is lost because insufficient water is added |
| | Regular desludging required, and sludge needs careful handling |
| | Permeable soil required to dispose of effluent |

## Removal systems for excreta

### Overhung latrine

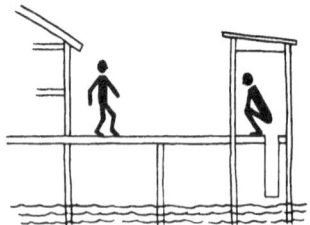

A latrine built over the sea, a river, or other body of water into which excreta drop directly, is known as an overhung latrine. If there is a strong current in the water the excreta are carried away. Local communities should be warned of the danger to health resulting from contact with or use of water into which excreta have been discharged.

| Advantages | Disadvantages |
|---|---|
| May be the only feasible system for communities living over water | Serious health risks |
| Cheap | |

### Bucket latrine

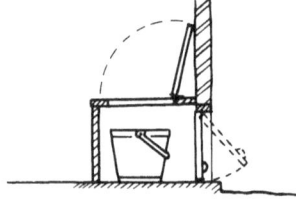

This latrine has a bucket or other container for the retention of faeces (and sometimes urine and anal cleaning material), which is periodically removed for treatment or disposal. Excreta removed in this way are sometimes termed nightsoil.

| Advantages | Disadvantages |
|---|---|
| Low initial cost | Malodorous |
| | Creates fly nuisance |
| | Danger to health of those who collect or use the nightsoil |
| | Collection is environmentally and physically undesirable |

### Vaults and cesspits

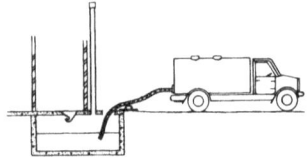

In some areas, watertight tanks called vaults are built under or close to latrines to store excreta until they are removed by hand (using buckets or similar receptacles) or by vacuum tanker. Similarly, household sewage may be stored in larger tanks called cesspits, which are usually emptied by vacuum tankers. Vaults or cesspits may be emptied when they are nearly full or on a regular basis.

| Advantages | Disadvantages |
|---|---|
| Satisfactory for users where there is a reliable and safe collection service | High construction and collection costs |
| | Removal by hand has even greater health risks than bucket latrines |
| | Irregular collection can lead to tanks overflowing |
| | Efficient infrastructure required |

## Sewerage

Discharge from WCs and other liquid wastes flow along a system of sewers to treatment works or directly into the sea or a river.

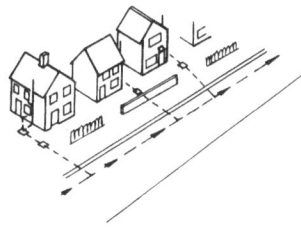

| Advantages | Disadvantages |
|---|---|
| User has no concern with what happens after the WC is flushed | High construction costs |
| No nuisance near the household | Efficient infrastructure required for construction, operation and maintenance |
| Treated effluent can be used for irrigation | Ample and reliable piped water supply required (a minimum of 70 litres per person per day is recommended) |
| | If discharge is to a water-course, adequate treatment required to avoid pollution |

Sewers of smaller diameter than usual (small-bore sewerage), sewers built nearer to the surface than usual, and sewers with flatter gradient than usual have been tried. Many of these systems require a chamber at each house to retain solids, which have to be removed and disposed of from time to time. Some of these systems have been found to be suitable for providing sanitation simultaneously for a large number of high-density dwellings.

PART II
# Detailed design, construction, operation and maintenance

CHAPTER 5
# Technical factors affecting excreta disposal

## Human wastes

### Volume of fresh human wastes

The amount of faeces and urine excreted daily by individuals varies considerably depending on water consumption, climate, diet and occupation. The only way to obtain an accurate determination of the amount at a particular location is direct measurement. Table 5.1 shows some reported average quantities of faeces excreted by adults (grams per person per day).

Even in comparatively homogeneous groups there may be a wide variation in the amounts of excreta produced. For example, Egbunwe (1980) reported a range of 500–900 g of faeces per person per day in eastern Nigeria. Generally, active adults eating a high-fibre diet and living in a rural area produce more faeces than children or elderly people living in urban areas eating a low-fibre diet. Both Shaw (1962) and Pradt (1971) suggested that the total amount of excreta is about one litre per person per day.

The amount of urine is greatly dependent on temperature and humidity, commonly ranging from 0.6 to 1.1 litres per person per day.

In the absence of local information the following figures are suggested as reasonable averages:

— high-protein diet in a temperate climate: faeces 120 g, urine 1.2 l, per person per day.
— vegetarian diet in a tropical climate: faeces 400 g, urine 1.0 l, per person per day.

**Table 5.1. Quantity of wet faeces excreted by adults (in grams per person per day)**

| Place | Quantity | Reference |
|---|---|---|
| China (men) | 209 | Scott (1952) |
| India | 255 | Macdonald (1952) |
| India | 311 | Tandon & Tandon (1975) |
| Peru (rural Indians) | 325 | Crofts (1975) |
| Uganda (villagers) | 470 | Burkitt et al. (1974) |
| Malaysia (rural) | 477 | Balasegaram & Burkitt (1976) |
| Kenya | 520 | Cranston & Burkitt (1975) |

## Decomposition of faeces and urine

As soon as excreta are deposited they start to decompose, eventually becoming a stable material with no unpleasant smell and containing valuable plant nutrients. During decomposition the following processes take place.

- Complex organic compounds, such as proteins and urea, are broken down into simpler and more stable forms.
- Gases such as ammonia, methane, carbon dioxide and nitrogen are produced and released into the atmosphere.
- Soluble material is produced which may leach into the underlying or surrounding soil or be washed away by flushing water or groundwater.
- Pathogens are destroyed because they are unable to survive in the environment of the decomposing material.

The decomposition is mainly carried out by bacteria although fungi and other organisms may assist. The bacterial activity may be either aerobic, i.e., taking place in the presence of air or free oxygen (for example, following defecation and urination on to the ground), or anaerobic, i.e., in an environment containing no air or free oxygen (for example, in a septic tank or at the bottom of a pit). In some situations both aerobic and anaerobic conditions may apply in turn. When all available oxygen has been used by aerobic bacteria, facultative bacteria capable of either aerobic or anaerobic activity take over, and finally anaerobic organisms commence activity.

Pathogens may be destroyed because the temperature and moisture content of the decomposing material create hostile conditions. For example, during composting of a mixture of faeces and vegetable waste under fully aerobic conditions, the temperature may rise to 70 °C, which is too hot for the survival of intestinal organisms. Pathogens may also be attacked by predatory bacteria and protozoa, or may lose a contest for limited nutrients.

## Volumes of decomposed human wastes

As excreta become decomposed they are reduced in volume and mass owing to:

— evaporation of moisture;
— production of gases which usually escape to the atmosphere;
— leaching of soluble substances;
— transport of insoluble material by the surrounding liquids;
— consolidation at the bottom of pits and tanks under the weight of superimposed solids and liquids.

Little information is available regarding the rate at which the reduction takes place although there are indications that temperature is an important factor (Mara & Sinnatamby, 1986). Weibel et al. (1949)

**Fig. 5.1. Rate of accumulation of sludge and scum in 205 septic tanks in the United States of America (from Weibel et al., 1949)**

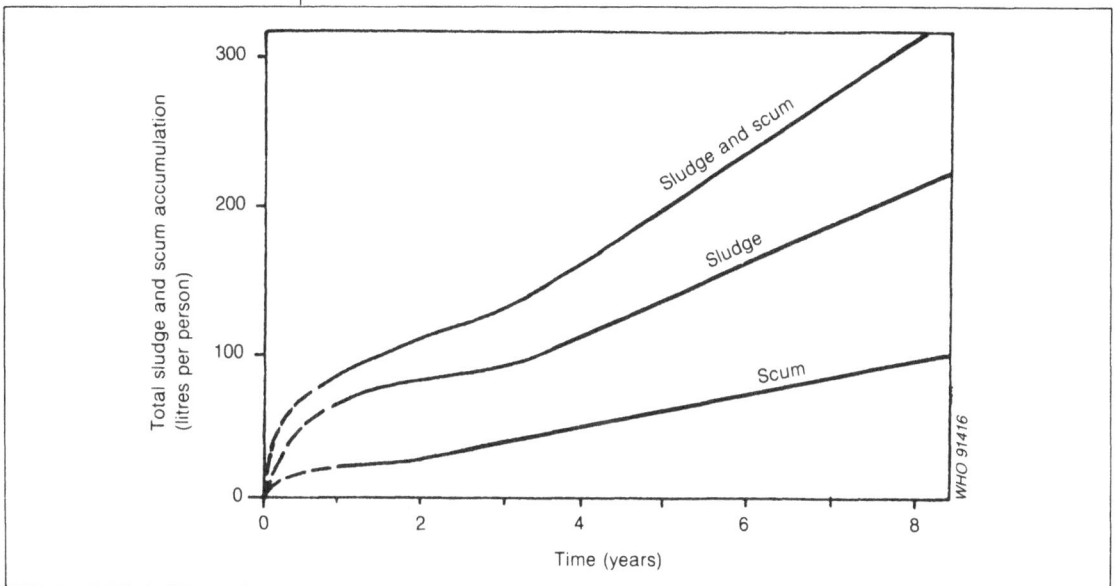

**Table 5.2. Excreta accumulation rates (litres per person per year)**

| Location | Accumulated excreta | Remarks | Reference |
|---|---|---|---|
| Zimbabwe | 20 | Latrine regularly washed down; degradable cleaning material | Morgan & Mara (1982) |
| West Bengal | 25 | Wet pit—ablution water used | Wagner & Lanoix (1958) |
| West Bengal | 34 | Wet pit | Baskaran (1962) |
| Philippines | 40 | Wet pit; degradable cleaning material | Wagner & Lanoix (1958) |
| USA | 42 | Faeces (adult); half amount for children | Geyer et al. (1968) |
| Brazil | 47 | Dry pit | Sanches & Wagner (1954) |
| Philippines | 60 | Dry pit; degradable cleaning material | Wagner & Lanoix (1958) |

measured the sludge accumulation rate in 205 septic tanks in the United States of America, and obtained the results shown in Fig. 5.1; other authors have reported the accumulation rates listed in Table 5.2.

The factors with the biggest effect on the sludge accumulation rate are whether decomposition takes place above or below the water table and the type of anal cleaning material used. Decomposition under water produces a much greater reduction in volume than decomposition in air. This is due to better consolidation, more rapid decomposition and removal of the finer material in the water flow. Anal cleaning

**Table 5.3. Suggested maximum sludge accumulation rates (litres per person per year)**

|  | Sludge accumulation rate |
| --- | --- |
| Wastes retained in water where degradable anal cleaning materials are used | 40 |
| Wastes retained in water where non-degradable anal cleaning materials are used | 60 |
| Waste retained in dry conditions where degradable anal cleaning materials are used | 60 |
| Wastes retained in dry conditions where non-degradable anal cleaning materials are used | 90 |

materials vary widely around the world, from those requiring little or no storage space, such as water, to those having a greater volume than the excreta, such as corn cobs, cement bags or stones.

When designing a latrine it is strongly recommended that local sludge accumulation rates should be measured. In the absence of local data, the volumes given in Table 5.3 are suggested as a maximum. There is some evidence to indicate that these figures are on the high side. However, if refuse is added to excreta, the accumulation rate may be much greater.

Where excreta are stored for short periods only, such as in double pit latrines or composting toilets, the reduction process may not be complete before the sludge is removed. In such cases it will be necessary to use higher sludge accumulation rates than indicated above. A 50% increase is tentatively suggested.

## Ground conditions

Ground conditions affect the selection and design of sanitation systems, and the following five factors should be taken into consideration:

— bearing capacity of the soil;
— self-supporting properties of the pits against collapse;
— depth of excavation possible;
— infiltration rate;
— groundwater pollution risk.

### Bearing capacity of the soil

All structures require foundations, and some soils are suitable only for lightweight materials because of their poor load-carrying capacity— marshy and peaty soils are obvious examples. In general, it is safe to assume that if the ground is suitable for building a house it will be strong enough to support the weight of a latrine superstructure made of similar materials, providing the pit is appropriately lined.

## Self-supporting properties of the pits

Many types of latrine require the excavation of a pit. Unless there is specific evidence to the contrary (i.e., an existing unlined shallow well that has not collapsed), it is recommended that all pits should be lined to their full depth. Many soils may appear to be self-supporting when first excavated, particularly cohesive soils, such as clays and silts, and naturally bonded soils, such as laterites and soft rock. These self-supporting properties may well be lost over time owing to changes in the moisture content or decomposition of the bonding agent through contact with air and/or moisture. It is almost impossible to predict when these changes are likely to occur or even if they will occur at all. It is therefore safer to line the pit. The lining should permit liquid to percolate into the surrounding soil.

## Depth of excavation

Loose ground, hard rock or groundwater near to the surface limit the depth of excavation possible using simple hand tools. Large rocks may be broken if a fire is lit around them and then cold water poured on the hot rock. Excavation below the water table and in loose ground is possible by "caissoning" (see Chapter 7), but it is expensive and not usually suitable for use by householders building their own latrines.

## Infiltration rate

The soil type affects the rate at which liquid infiltrates from pits and drainage trenches. Clays that expand when wet may become impermeable. Other soils such as silts and fine sands may be permeable to clean water but become blocked when transmitting effluent containing suspended and dissolved solids.

Opinions vary regarding the areas through which infiltration takes place. For example, Lewis et al. (1980) recommended that only the base of pits or drainage trenches should be considered and that lateral movement (the sidewall influence) be ignored. Mara (1985b) and others have assumed that infiltration takes place only through the side walls as the base rapidly becomes blocked with sludge. Until more evidence is available, it is recommended that the design of pits and trenches should be based on infiltration through the side walls up to the maximum liquid level. For trenches, the area of both walls should be used.

The rate of infiltration also depends on the level of the groundwater table relative to the liquid in the pit or trench. In the unsaturated zone, the flow of liquid is induced by gravity and cohesive and adhesive forces set up in the soil. Seasonal variation may produce a change in the amount of air and water in the soil pores and this will affect the flow rate. Conditions at the end of the wet season should normally be used for design purposes as this is usually the time when the groundwater level is at its highest. In the saturated zone all pores are filled with water and drainage depends on the size of the pores and the difference in level between the liquid in the pit or trench and the surrounding groundwater.

Soil porosity also affects infiltration. Soils with large pores, such as sand and gravel, and rocks such as some sandstones and those containing fissures, drain easily. Silt and clay soils, however, have very small pores and tend to retain water. Soils containing organic materials also tend to retain water but the roots of plants and trees break up the soil, producing holes through which liquids can drain quickly.

The rate of groundwater flow in unsaturated soils is a complex function of the size, shape and distribution of the pores and fissures, the soil chemistry and the presence of air. The speed of flow is normally less than 0.3 m per day except in fissured rocks and coarse gravels, where the speed may be more than 5.0 m per day, with increased likelihood of groundwater pollution.

### Pore clogging

Soil pores eventually become clogged by effluent from pits or drainage trenches. This may reduce or even stop infiltration through the soil. Clogging may be caused by:

— blockage of pores by solids filtered from the liquid;
— growth of microorganisms and their wastes;
— swelling of clay minerals; and
— precipitation of insoluble salts.

When liquid first infiltrates into unsaturated soil, aerobic bacteria decompose much of the organic matter filtered from the liquid, keeping the pores clear for the passage of air as well as effluent. However, once organic matter builds up so that air cannot pass through the pores, the rate of decomposition (now by anaerobic bacteria) is slower, and heavy black deposits of insoluble sulfides are built up.

Clogging of the pores can be minimized by ensuring that infiltration occurs uniformly over the whole system. Poorly designed infiltration systems (particularly trenches) often cause the liquid to converge on a small section of the system. This produces localized high infiltration rates and clogging in that area. Clogging can sometimes be reduced by a regime of alternate "resting" and "dosing" of the soil. The infiltration area is allowed to rest, i.e., to become fully drained of liquid for a period before infiltration recommences. During the resting period, air reaches the soil surface and the anaerobic bacteria causing the clogging die off, allowing the surface to become unclogged.

### Determining infiltration rates

It is rarely possible to measure accurately the rate of flow of effluent from pits and drainage trenches, especially as the flow often decreases as soil pores become clogged. Consequently various empirical rules are used. Some recommendations are based on the rate of percolation of clean water from trial holes dug on the site of a proposed pit or drainage field using various design criteria to allow for differences in infiltration rates (US Department of Health, Education, and Welfare, 1969; British Standards Institution, 1972). Laak et al. (1974) found that, for a wide range of soils, the infiltration rates of effluent were 10–30 litres per m² per day. A conservative rate of 10 litres per m² per day was recommended for general application. On the other hand, rates of up to 200 litres per m² per day are considered applicable in practice in the United States of America (US Department of Health, Education, and Welfare, 1969), and Aluko (1977) found that, in Nigeria, designs with a maximum of 294 litres per m² per day have proved satisfactory. The infiltration capacities given in Table 5.4 (US Environmental Protection Agency, 1980) are recommended as a basis for the sizing of pits and drainage trenches where information about actual infiltration rates is not available. The capacities given for coarse soils are restricted to prevent possible groundwater pollution and therefore may be unnecessarily conservative in areas where this is not a problem. Gravel is capable of much higher infiltration rates, which may be a problem in areas where shallow groundwater is used for human consumption. This pollution problem can be reduced by the provision of a sand envelope as described on pp. 40–41.

**Table 5.4. Recommended infiltration capacities**[a]

| Type of soil | Infiltration capacity, settled sewage (l per m² per day) |
| --- | --- |
| Coarse or medium sand | 50 |
| Fine sand, loamy sand | 33 |
| Sandy loam, loam | 25 |
| Porous silty clay and porous silty clay loam | 20 |
| Compact silty loam, compact silty clay loam and non-expansive clay | 10 |
| Expansive clay | < 10 |

[a]Source: US Environmental Protection Agency, 1980.

## Groundwater pollution risk

This section summarizes the likely effects of on-site sanitation systems on groundwater and the ways in which pollution can be minimized. Lewis et al. (1980) have carried out detailed reviews of these aspects.

The effluent from pits and drainage trenches may contain pathogens and chemical substances that could contaminate drinking-water supplies. Because of their comparatively large size, protozoa and helminths are rapidly removed by the straining action of the soil, but bacteria and viruses are more persistent. The bacterial and viral pathogens that may be carried in water are discussed in Chapter 2.

Of the chemical substances generally present in domestic wastes, only nitrates present serious health dangers. Young babies bottle-fed with milk made from water with a high nitrate concentration may develop "blue baby disease", methaemoglobinaemia, which can be fatal if untreated. There is conflicting evidence suggesting that low nitrate concentrations may contribute to gastric cancer (Nitrate Co-ordination Group, 1986).

The usual means by which effluents affect drinking-water supplies is through pollution of groundwater that feeds wells and boreholes. A further danger is when effluent infiltrates the ground at shallow depth near to water pipes in which there is intermittent flow or in which the pressure is at times very low. Just as poor joints, cracks and holes in the pipe walls allow water to leak out when the pipes are full, so effluent leaks into the pipes when they are empty or under reduced pressure. Recommendations for allowable levels of pollutants in drinking-water are given in *Guidelines for drinking-water quality* (WHO, 1984).

### Purification in unsaturated soil

Effluent passing through unsaturated soil (that is, soil above the groundwater table) is purified by filtration and by biological and adsorption processes. Filtration is most effective in the organic mat where the soil pores are clogged. In sandy soils, Butler et al. (1954) found a dramatic reduction in coliforms in the first 50 mm. The passage of pollutants from a new pit or drainage trench reduces as the pores become clogged.

Viruses, because of their small size, are little affected by filtration and their removal is almost entirely by adsorption on to the surface of soil particles; this is greatest where the pH is low (Stumm & Morgan, 1981). Adsorption of both viruses and bacteria is greatest in soils with a high clay content, and is favoured by a long residence time—that is, when flow rates are slow. Because the flow is much slower in the unsaturated zone than below the groundwater table, there is longer contact between soil and effluent there, increasing opportunities for adsorption. Adsorbed microorganisms can be dislodged, for example by flushes of effluent or following heavy rainfall, and may then pass into lower strata of the soil.

Viruses, whether they have been removed or remain in effluent, live longer at lower temperatures (Yeager & O'Brien, 1979). Both viruses and bacteria live longer in moist conditions than in dry conditions, and therefore in soils with a good water-holding capacity than in sandy soils. Bacteria live longer in alkaline than in acid soils. They also survive well in soils containing organic material, where there may be some regrowth.

Generally there is little risk of groundwater pollution where there is at least 2 m of relatively fine soil between a pit or drainage trench and the water table, providing the rate of application is not greater than 50 mm/day (equivalent to 50 litres per m² per day). This distance may have to be increased in areas subject to intense rainfall, as the increased infiltration rate produced by the percolating rainwater may carry pollution further.

Fissures in consolidated rock may allow rapid flow of effluent to underlying groundwater with little removal of microorganisms. Holes in soil caused by tree roots or burrowing animals can act in the same way as fissures.

### *Purification in groundwater*

There is little information about survival of either viruses or bacteria in groundwater, although it appears that low temperature favours long survival times. Enteric bacteria may survive in cool groundwater for more than three months (Kibbey et al., 1978). Field experiments indicate that the maximum distance that viruses and bacteria travel in groundwater before being destroyed is equal to the distance travelled by the groundwater in about ten days (Lewis et al., 1980).

In fine-grained soils and pollution sources surrounded by a mature organic mat, the distance travelled may be as little as 3 m, whereas a new source in fast-flowing groundwater may cause pollution up to 25 m downstream (Caldwell, 1937). The pollution extends from the source in the direction of groundwater flow, with only limited vertical and horizontal dispersion. However, this does not apply to pollution in fissured ground, where the pollution may flow through the fissures for several hundred metres, often in an unpredictable direction.

In most cases the commonly used figure of a minimum of 15 m between a pollution source and a downstream water abstraction point will be satisfactory. Where the abstraction point is not downstream of the pollution, i.e., to the side or upstream, the distance can be reduced provided that the groundwater is not abstracted at such a rate that its direction of flow is turned towards the abstraction point (Fig. 5.2). This is particularly useful in densely populated communities, where shallow groundwater is used as a water supply.

If it is not possible to provide sufficient space between the latrine and the water point, consideration should be given to extracting water from a lower level in the aquifer (Fig. 5.3). The predominant flow of groundwater (except fissured flow) is along the strata, with very little vertical movement. Provided the extraction rate is not too great (handpump or bucket extraction is acceptable), and the well is properly sealed where it passes through the pollution zone, there should be little or no risk of pollution.

**Fig. 5.2. Zone of pollution from pit latrine**

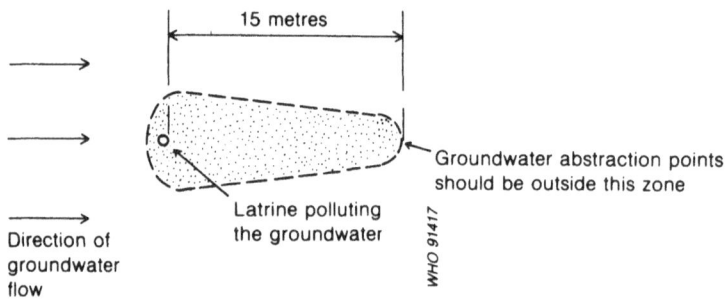

**Fig. 5.3. Protecting a hand pump from the pollution from a pit latrine**

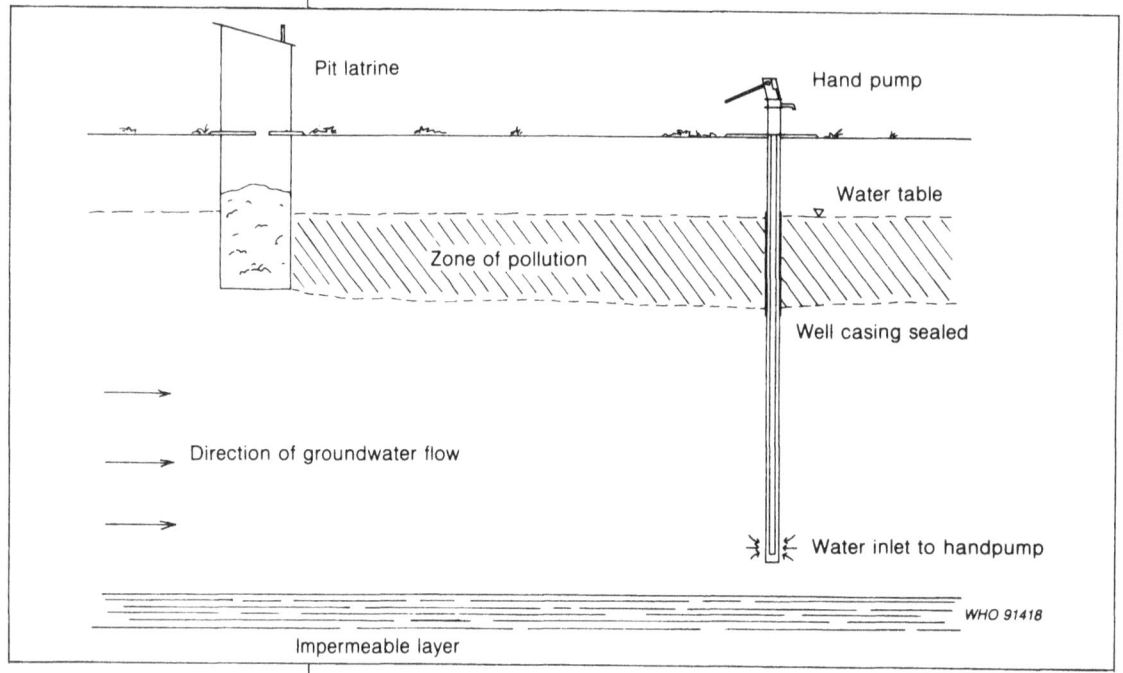

### Significance of pollution

While faecal pollution of drinking-water should be avoided, the dangers of groundwater pollution from on-site sanitation should not be exaggerated. A depth of two metres of unsaturated sandy or loamy soil below a pit or drainage trench is likely to provide an effective barrier to groundwater pollution and there may be little lateral spread of pollu-

**Fig. 5.4. Reducing the pollution from a pit latrine with a barrier of sand**

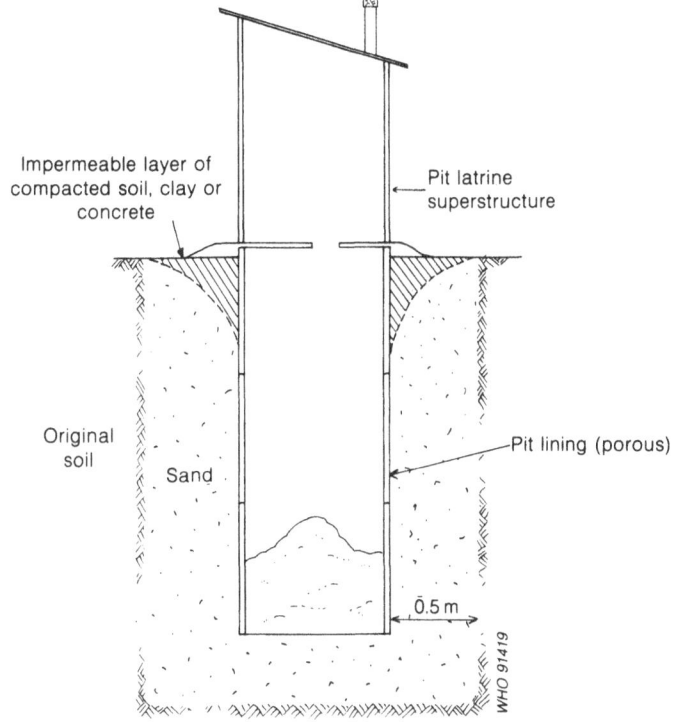

tion. Where the groundwater is shallow, artificial barriers of sand around pits can control pollution (Fig. 5.4).

Unless water is extracted locally for domestic purposes, pollution of groundwater from on-site sanitation does no harm and is to be preferred to the considerable risks associated with defecation in the open. Where on-site sanitation would result in pollution of wells used for drinking-water, it is generally cheaper and easier to provide water from outside than to build sewers or use vacuum tankers to remove excreta.

## Insect and vermin problems

### Insects

Many insects are attracted to excreta because they provide rich organic material and water, both of which are essential for the insects' development. The most important groups from a health point of view are mosquitos, houseflies, blowflies and cockroaches.

### Mosquitos

Some mosquitos, particularly *Culex pipiens* and some species of *Anopheles*, breed in polluted water, including that found in some pit latrines. Unlike flies, mosquitos are not deterred by low light levels, so keeping excreta in a dark place does not prevent them from breeding. Possible solutions are to keep the pit fully sealed or to cover the surface of the liquid with a film that prevents mosquito larvae from breathing. Oil and proprietary chemicals have been used effectively but may contaminate the groundwater. An alternative is to use small plastic balls that float on the surface producing a mechanical cover to the liquid. Fortunately many latrines only have a free water surface for a short period immediately after starting up or emptying. After that a layer of scum forms on the water surface preventing further mosquito breeding.

### Houseflies and blowflies

These are medium- to large-sized flies that are attracted to human food as well as faeces and refuse. The three larval stages are found in excreta or mixtures of excreta and decaying vegetable matter. Solid, moist and fermenting material is most suitable for the breeding of houseflies, but the larvae of the blowfly prefer more liquid faeces and may liquefy masses of faecal material (Feachem et al., 1983). Open pit latrines are ideal breeding places.

Flies use both sight and smell to find food. This is an important consideration when designing latrines since not only must excreta be stored in a dark place but any ventilation holes must be screened.

### Cockroaches

Cockroaches are attracted to latrines by the moisture and organic matter; they are then likely to transmit disease by carrying pathogenic organisms on their bodies. Provided that a site has a continuous food supply the cockroaches tend to remain where they are. Accordingly latrines should be sited as far as possible from where food is stored and prepared, to prevent migration of cockroaches from one to the other.

## Rats

Rats look upon excreta as a food source. If they come in contact with excreta and then with food intended for human consumption there is a possibility of their transmitting disease. In Nepal, there has been a problem with rats burrowing into double-pit latrines through the holes left in the pit walls. Not only does this create a possible transmission route for disease but the rats deposit large volumes of soil in the pit which rapidly fill it. A full lining of the top 0.5–1.0 m of any pit should prevent rats from entering.

# CHAPTER 6

# Operation and maintenance of on-site sanitation

Any review of on-site sanitation shows that there are a large number of options to choose from. This is to be expected, since every project has different characteristics, requiring a different solution. Many of the alternatives are variations on, or combinations of, other designs and it is not possible to describe them all. Those planning on-site sanitation should adopt and combine the major options described in any way that will produce the most appropriate solution.

This chapter describes how the different types of latrine introduced in Chapter 4 work and discusses their relative merits. Details of construction of individual parts is given in Chapter 7 and design examples in Chapter 8.

## Pit latrines

The principle of all types of pit latrine is that wastes such as excreta, anal cleaning materials, sullage and refuse are deposited in a hole in the ground. The liquids percolate into the surrounding soil and the organic material decomposes producing:

— gases such as carbon dioxide and methane, which are liberated to the atmosphere or disperse into the surrounding soil;
— liquids, which percolate into the surrounding soil;
— a decomposed and consolidated residue.

In one form or another, pit latrines are widely used in most developing countries. The health benefits and convenience depend upon the quality of the design, construction and maintenance. At worst, pit latrines that are badly designed, constructed and maintained provide foci for the transmission of disease and may be no better than indiscriminate defecation. At best, they provide a standard of sanitation that is at least as good as other more sophisticated methods.

Simplicity of operation and construction, low construction costs, the fact that they can be built by householders with a minimum of external assistance, and effectiveness in breaking the routes by which diseases are spread, are among the advantages that make pit latrines the most practical form of sanitation available to many people. This is especially true where there is no reliable, continuous and ample piped water supply.

Unfortunately, past failures, especially of public facilities, discourage some sanitation field workers from advocating their widespread use. Objections to the use of pit latrines are that poorly designed and poorly constructed latrines produce unpleasant smells, that they are associated with the breeding of undesirable insects (particularly flies, mosquitos and cockroaches), that they are liable to collapse, and that they may produce chemical and biological contamination of groundwater. Pit latrines that are well designed, sited and constructed, and are properly used need not have any of these faults.

## Design life

As a general rule, pits should be designed to last as long as possible. Pits designed to last 25–30 years are not uncommon and a design life of 15–20 years is perfectly reasonable. The longer a pit lasts, the lower will be the average annual economic cost and the greater the social benefits from the original input.

In some areas, ground conditions make it impractical to achieve such a design life. If the maximum possible design life is less than ten years, serious consideration should be given to using an alternating double-pit system. In such systems the pits must have a minimum life of two years. In the past, a minimum life of one year was considered sufficient for ensuring the death of most pathogenic organisms, but it is now known that an appreciable number of organisms can live longer (see Chapter 2). In any event the increased cost of designing a pit to last two years as compared to one designed to last one year is minimal because of decomposition and consolidation of the first year's sludge (see Chapter 5).

## Pit shape

The depth of the pit to some extent affects the plan shape. Deep pits (deeper than about 1.5 m) are usually circular, whereas shallow pits are commonly square or rectangular. As the pit gets deeper the load applied to the pit lining by the ground increases. At shallow depths, normal pit linings (concrete, brick masonry, etc.) are usually strong enough to support the soil without a detailed design. Also square or rectangular linings are easier to construct. At greater depths, the circular shape is structurally more stable and able to carry additional loading.

Commonly, pits are 1.0–1.5 m wide or in diameter, since this is a convenient size for a person to work inside during excavation. The cover slab required is simple to design and construct, and cheap to build.

## Emptying pits

The emptying of single pits containing fresh excreta presents problems because of the active pathogens in the sludge. In rural areas, where land availability is not a constraint, it is often advisable to dig another pit for a new latrine. The original pit may then be left for several years and when the second is filled it may be simplest to re-dig the first pit rather than to excavate a new hole in hard ground. The sludge will not cause any health problems and is beneficial as a fertilizer. However, in urban areas, where it is not possible to excavate further holes and where the investment in pit-lining and superstructure has been substantial, the pit must be emptied.

From the public health point of view, manual removal should be avoided. Where the groundwater level is so high that the pit is flooded or where the pit is sealed and fitted with an effluent overflow, the wet sludge can be removed by ordinary vacuum tankers. These tankers are the same as those used for emptying septic tanks or road gullies (Fig. 6.1). Hand-powered diaphragm pumps have so far proved to be very slow and laborious in emptying pits and have not been widely adopted.

Where pits are mainly dry, the greater part of the contents will have consolidated into solid material which conventional vacuum tankers cannot lift. In addition to this difficulty Boesch & Schertenleib (1985) summarized pit emptying problems as follows.

● The machinery may be too large to get to the latrines. Conventional vacuum trucks are too big to be driven into the centre of many ancient cities or urban/periurban unplanned or squatter settlements where pedestrian routes predominate.
● Maintenance of vacuum tankers is often poor. Their engines must be kept running all day, either to move the truck or to operate the pump when stationary. This causes rapid wear and makes them particularly susceptible to breakdown if preventive maintenance is neglected.

**Fig. 6.1. Vacuum tanker desludging a septic tank**

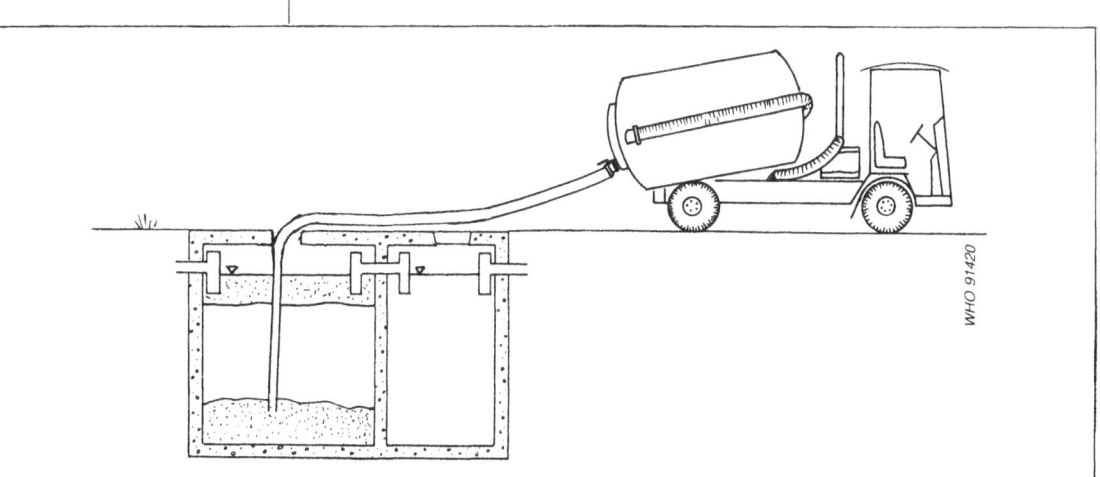

● Management and supervision of emptying services is often in-effective.

High-performance vacuum tankers able to deal with consolidated pit latrine sludge have been developed (Caroll, 1985; Boesch & Schertenleib, 1985) and are able to exhaust sludge over a horizontal distance of 60 m, thereby getting round problems of accessibility. However, considerable time is needed to set up and then dismantle and wash out the suction pipes.

As an alternative, the pump and tank may be mounted on a small, highly manoeuvrable site vehicle or on separate small vehicles in order to reach a latrine with limited accessibility. The disadvantage of using a smaller tank is that more journeys to the disposal point are required. Consequently, the suction pump is unused during this waiting period unless several small tankers are used with each pump. This can lead to a considerable increase in costs, particularly where disposal points are distant from the latrines. Larger-capacity transfer tankers may be employed to ensure best use of the costly vacuum pump.

Another approach involves the use of a container which can be manhandled close to an otherwise inaccessible latrine, even through the house where necessary. Small-diameter, clean vacuum lines connect the container to the distant tanker, providing the suction necessary to fill the container (Fig. 6.2). A fail-safe method of shutting off the sludge intake when the container is full is required to prevent sludge being carried through the air-line into the vacuum filter and

**Fig. 6.2. Remote vacuum pump emptying system**

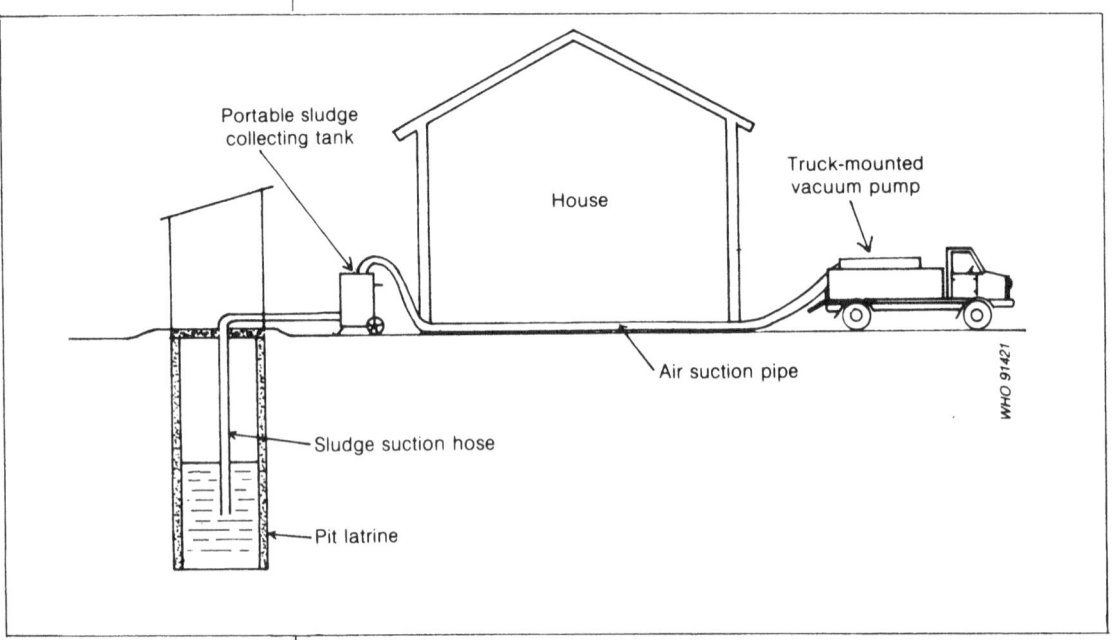

engine. The containers have to be of such a size that they can be manhandled safely when full but also that the least possible number of container movements is required for each pit (Wilson, 1987).

All these systems are relatively expensive and require efficient mechanical maintenance to ensure reliability. The least sophisticated system should be used wherever possible for the majority of pit emptyings.

## Simple pit latrines

The simple pit latrine (Fig. 6.3) consists of a hole in the ground (which may be wholly or partially lined) covered by a squatting slab or seat where the user defecates. The defecation hole may be provided with a cover or plug to prevent the entrance of flies or egress of odour while the pit is not being used.

The cover slab is commonly surrounded by some form of super-structure that provides shelter and privacy for the user. The super-structure design is irrelevant to the operation of the latrine but crucial to the acceptability of the latrine to the user. Superstructures range from a simple shelter of sacks or sticks to a building of bricks or blocks costing more than the rest of the latrine. The choice of superstructure will reflect the income and customs of the user.

**Fig. 6.3. Simple pit latrine**

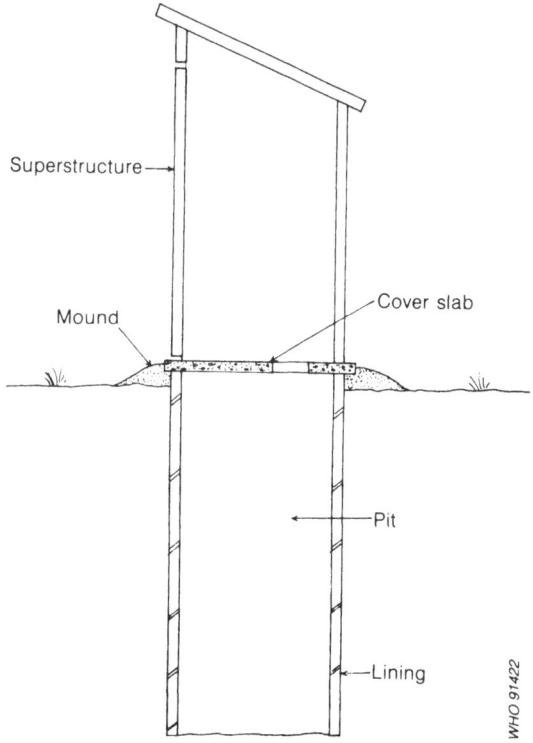

The cover slab should be raised at least 150 mm above the surrounding ground to divert surface water away from the pit. Commonly, the cover slab sits directly on the lining, but if the lining is made of very thin material, such as an old oil drum, a concrete foundation beam may be necessary to distribute the load of the slab to the lining and surrounding ground (Fig. 6.4).

The simple pit latrine is the cheapest form of sanitation possible. Once constructed it requires very little attention other than keeping the latrine area clean and ensuring that the hole cover is in place when the latrine is not in use. Unfortunately the superstructure frequently becomes infested with flies and mosquitos and full of pungent odours because users do not replace the squat hole cover after use. Self-closing hole covers have been tried but are often disliked because the cover rests against the user's back. There may also be resistance to constructing new simple pit latrines because of their resemblance to existing, badly constructed, pit latrines.

## Ventilated pit latrines

These are also known as ventilated improved pit (VIP) latrines (Fig. 6.5). The major nuisances that discourage the use of simple pit latrines—smell and flies—are reduced or eliminated through the incorporation of a vertical vent pipe with a flyscreen at the top (Morgan, 1977). Wind passing over the top of the vent pipe causes a flow of air from the pit through the vent pipe to the atmosphere and a

**Fig. 6.4. Ring beam on top of a thin pit lining to support the cover slab**

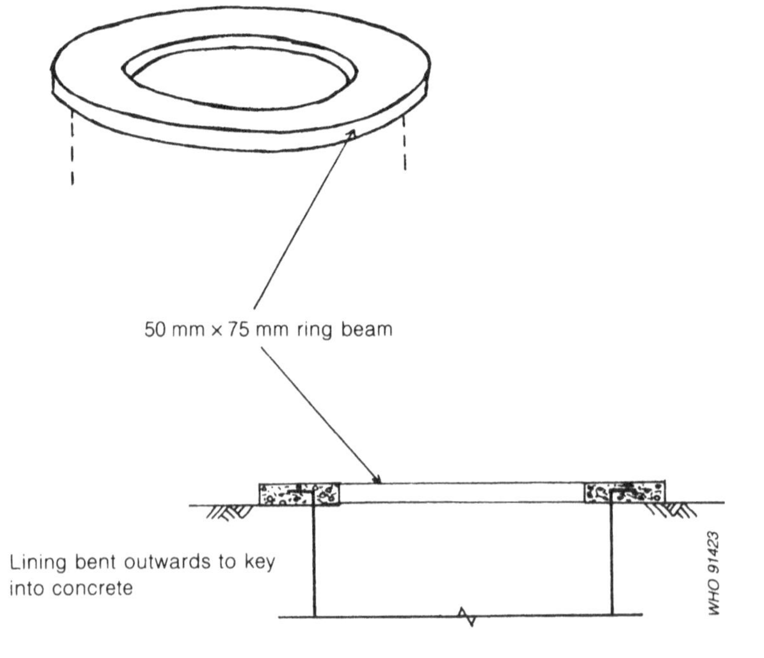

50 mm × 75 mm ring beam

Lining bent outwards to key into concrete

WHO 91423

**Fig. 6.5. Ventilated improved pit (VIP) latrine**

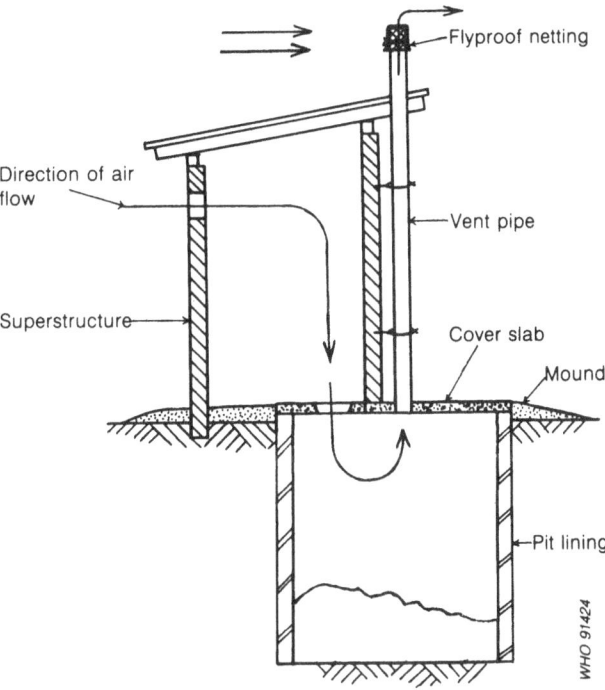

downdraught from the superstructure through the squat hole or seat into the pit. This continuous flow of air removes smells resulting from the decomposing excreta in the pit and vents the gases to the atmosphere at the top of the vent pipe rather than through the superstructure. The flow of air is increased if the doorway of the superstructure faces the prevailing wind (Mara, 1984). If a door is fitted it should be kept shut at all times (except when entering or leaving) to keep the inside of the latrine reasonably dark, but there should be a gap, normally above the door, for air to enter. The area of this gap should be at least three times the cross-sectional area of the vent pipe.

The superstructure can be constructed in the form of a spiral (Fig. 6.6). This excludes most of the light whether a door is fitted or not. The defecation hole must be left open to allow the free passage of air. The vent pipe should extend at least 50 cm above the latrine superstructure except where the latter has a conical roof, in which case the pipe should extend as high as the apex. Air turbulence caused by surrounding buildings or other obstructions may cause reverse air flow, leading to foul odours and flies in the superstructure. If mean wind speeds are about 2 m/s, as is fairly common in rural areas, air speeds in the vent pipe are about 1 m/s (Ryan & Mara, 1983). Air flow may also occur at lower wind speeds because of solar radiation heating the air in the vent pipe, causing the air to rise. The vent pipe should then be placed on the equator side of the superstructure. It may be

**Fig. 6.6. Spiral construction for the superstructure**

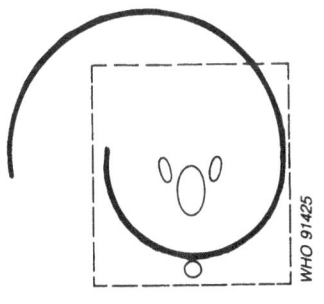

painted black to increase solar absorption, if the material of the pipe is not itself black.

In latrines relying on solar radiation for ventilation, foul odours are sometimes experienced in the superstructure at certain times of the day (usually early morning). This occurs where the outside air temperature is colder than the air in the pit, which may prevent the air circulating. Very little can be done to prevent this, other than sealing the defecation hole at night.

In addition to removing odours from the pit, the screened vent pipe significantly controls flies. In Zimbabwe, Morgan (1977) compared the number of flies leaving the squat hole of a VIP latrine with the number leaving a simple pit latrine. The results are shown in Table 6.1.

Flies are attracted to the pit by the odour coming from the vent pipe but are unable to enter because of the screen. A few flies enter the pit through the squat hole or seat, and lay eggs in the pit. New young flies attempt to leave the pit by flying towards the light. If the latrine superstructure is kept sufficiently dark, the major source of light is at the top of the vent pipe, but the screen prevents the flies from escaping there and they eventually fall back into the pit to die.

Well-constructed and maintained VIP latrines combat all the problems associated with simple pit latrines, except mosquitos. However, they are considerably more expensive than simple pits, since a ventilation pipe and full superstructure are required. Because the defecating hole is directly over the pit they accept any form of anal cleaning material without blocking. Routine operation is limited to keeping the superstructure clean, ensuring that the door (where fitted) is kept closed, occasionally checking that the fly-proof netting on top of the vent pipe is not blocked or broken, and pouring water down the vent pipe once a year to remove spiders' webs.

**Table 6.1. Comparison of the numbers of flies leaving the squat holes of a simple pit latrine and a VIP latrine[a]**

| Period of trapping | No. trapped in unvented privy | No. trapped in vented privy |
|---|---|---|
| 8 October–5 November | 1723 | 5 |
| 5 November–3 December | 5742 | 20 |
| 3–24 December | 6488 | 121 |

[a] Source: Morgan, 1977.

## Ventilated double-pit latrines

Although it is usually best to provide large deep pits, this may not be possible where rock or groundwater lie within one or two metres of the ground surface. A variation of the VIP latrine suitable for such situations has two shallow pits side by side under a single superstructure (Fig. 6.7). The pits are usually lined with bricks or blocks. Each

**Fig. 6.7. Double-pit VIP latrine**

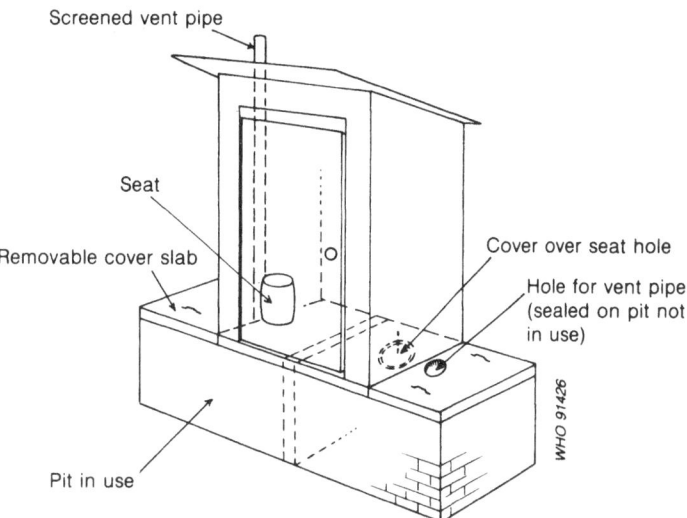

pit may have its own squat hole or seat. Alternatively, slabs may be movable, one with a hole for the pit in use and a plain slab for the other pit. Whichever design is used, only one hole must be available for defecation at any time. The latrine may be provided with two ventilation pipes (one for each pit) but more usually only one is fitted, to the pit in use. The hole for the ventilation pipe for the pit not in use is sealed. As with single VIP latrines, the superstructure must be kept partially dark at all times to discourage flies.

## Operation

One pit is used until it is filled to within about half a metre of the top. The defecation hole over the full pit is then sealed and the one over the empty pit opened. Where necessary, the ventilation pipe is moved from the full to the empty pit, and the vent hole in the slab of the full pit sealed. The second pit is then used until filled to within half a metre of the top. The contents of the first pit can now be removed and the pit reused. The pits must be large enough to allow each pit to be used for at least two years. This ensures that when the pit contents are dug out most of the pathogenic organisms have died.

Double-pit latrines can be considered as permanent installations. The small effective capacity (0.72 m³ for a family of six, using a sludge build-up rate of 60 litres per person per year, as suggested in Chapter 5) enables pits to be relatively shallow, and therefore easier to empty than deep pits. The pits should extend beyond the superstructure, either to the sides or at the back, with removable slabs for emptying. These slabs should be easy to lift, but should be sealed to prevent flies getting in or out. The central wall between the two pits should be made with full mortar joints and may be rendered with cement mortar on both sides.

As with the single-pit VIP latrine, the double-pit VIP latrine has the advantages of reduced smell and fly nuisance. Also the contents of the latrine dug out every two years or so are a valuable soil conditioner (see Annex 1). Double-pit VIP latrines are usually (but not always) more expensive than single-pit VIP latrines, and require a greater operational input from the user, particularly in changing over pits. Some societies have shown resistance to handling the decomposed contents of the pit but this can often be overcome with education and time. Allowing people to see (and handle) the contents of a pit as it is emptied is the strongest persuader for those concerned.

All projects involving the construction of double-pit latrines must allow for a prolonged support programme. Householders need to be reminded to change pits at the right time and should be assisted in doing so. This assistance will probably have to be available for at least the first two pit changes to ensure that the complete cycle is covered.

## Pour-flush latrines

The problems of flies, mosquitos and smell in simple pit latrines may be overcome simply and cheaply by the installation of a pan with a water seal in the defecating hole (Fig. 6.8). Chapter 7 gives details of the design and fabrication of water seals. The pan is cleared by pouring (or, better, throwing) a few litres of water into the pan after defecation. The amount of water used varies between one and four litres depending mainly on the pan and trap geometry. Pans requiring a small amount of water for flushing have the added advantage of reducing the risk of groundwater pollution. The flushing water does not have to be clean. If access to clean water is limited, laundry, bathing or any other similar water may be used.

Pour-flush latrines are most appropriate for people who use water for anal cleaning, and squat to defecate, but they have also proved popular in countries where other cleaning materials are common. However, there is a likelihood of blockage where solid materials such as hard paper or corncobs are put in the pan. The placing of solid cleaning materials in a container for separate disposal is not generally recommended unless careful attention can be given to the handling of the waste and sterilizing of the container. Blockage may also be caused by material used by menstruating women. This should be disposed of separately, e.g., by burying or burning. Efforts to clear blockages often result in damage to the water seal.

In most cases, because of the small quantity of water required for flushing, pour-flush latrines are suitable where water has to be carried to the latrine from a standpipe, well, or other water source. There is no justification for the belief that the pit should be ventilated to prevent the build up of gases. A vent pipe adds to the cost of the latrine and any gases produced easily percolate into the surrounding soil.

**Fig. 6.8. Pour-flush latrine**

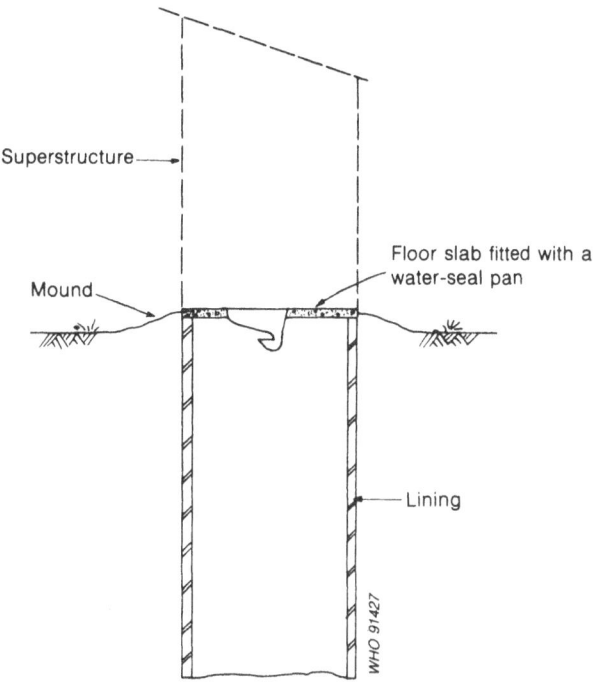

**Fig. 6.9. Offset pour-flush latrine**

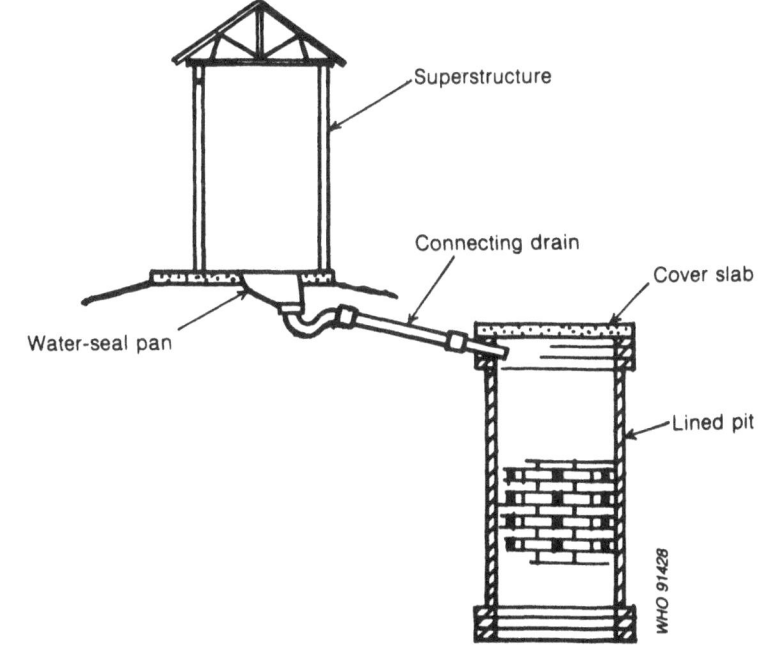

**Fig. 6.10. Brick-covered drain**

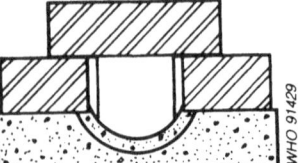

# Offset pour-flush latrines

An extension of the idea of the pour-flush pan with a water seal is for the pit to be outside the latrine building (Fig. 6.9). The contents of the pan are discharged through a short length of small-diameter pipe or covered channel with a minimum gradient of 1 in 30. PVC, concrete or clay pipes, 100 mm in diameter, are often used, but the diameter may be the same as the water seal (usually 65–85 mm). Masonry or brick-work channels with smooth circular concrete inverts have been adopted in some Asian countries. The channel is covered by precast concrete slabs or by bricks laid transversely across the top (Fig. 6.10). Pipes or channels should project at least 100 mm into the pit.

Generally speaking, an offset pour-flush latrine requires a larger volume of flushing water than a simple pour-flush latrine. The amount of water required depends on the pan design, pipe slope and roughness. As little as 1.5 litres has been recorded as necessary for each flush, but usually considerably more than this is required.

Offset pour-flush latrines are favoured by many because the super-structure can be permanent. When the pit is full, another pit can be dug alongside and the connecting pipe excavated and relaid to the new pit without damaging the superstructure (Fig. 6.11).

Another benefit is that the toilet can be located inside the house and the pit outside. If this layout is used, care must be taken to allow for movement of the pipe where it passes through the house wall. This can be achieved either by cutting a slot in the wall (Fig. 6.12) so that it does not bear directly on the pipe, or by installing two short lengths of pipe (Fig. 6.13) joining in the centre of the wall. Both systems allow movement of the wall without breaking the pipe. The distance of the

**Fig. 6.11. Moving the discharge pipe of an offset pour-flush latrine to a new pit**

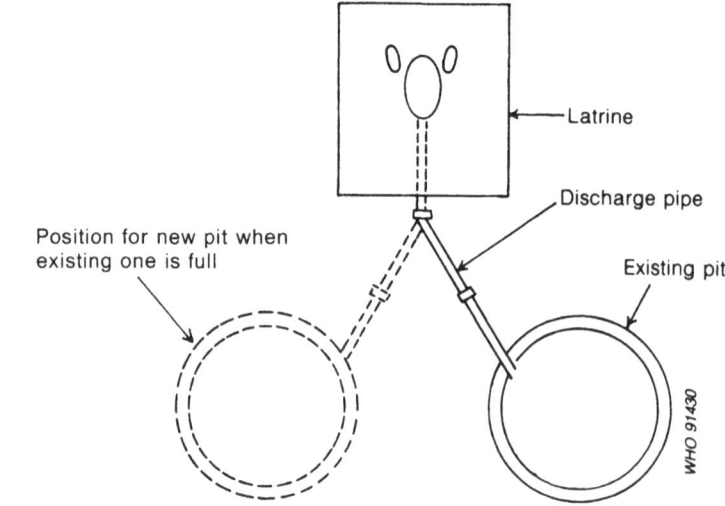

**Fig. 6.12. Pipe laid through a hole in an external wall**

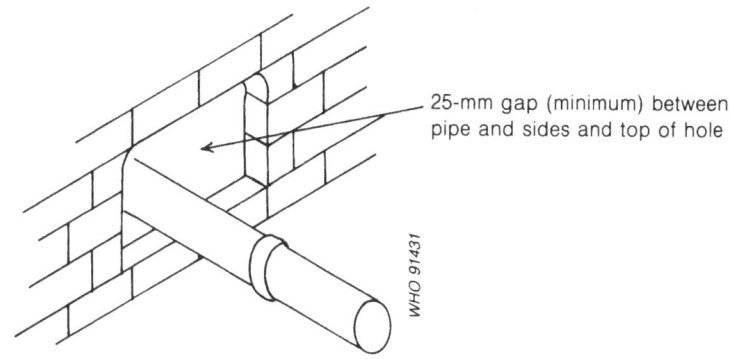

25-mm gap (minimum) between pipe and sides and top of hole

**Fig. 6.13. Pipe fixed in place through a wall**

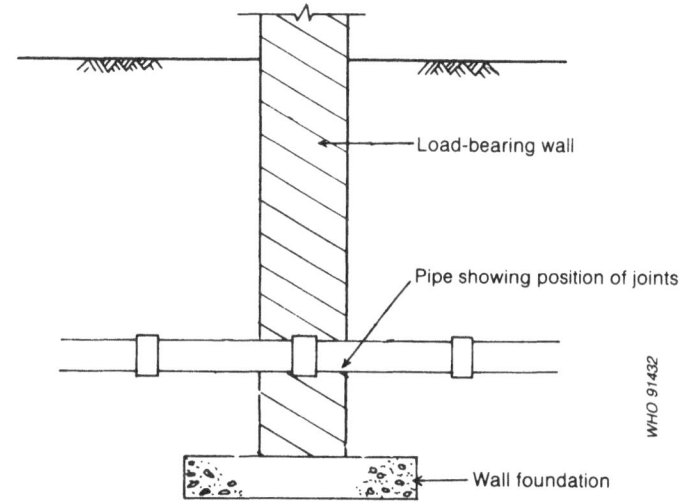

Load-bearing wall

Pipe showing position of joints

Wall foundation

pit from the house wall should be not less than its depth, to prevent the load from the wall causing the pit to collapse. If this is not possible, the pit may be located not less than one metre from the wall, provided that the pit is fully lined and the unsupported plan length parallel to the wall does not exceed one metre (Fig. 6.14).

## Double-pit offset pour-flush latrines

As with VIP latrines there are occasions when two shallow pits are more appropriate than a single deep pit. Double pits with pour-flush pans and water seals have been successfully used in India (Roy et al., 1984) and elsewhere. The pit design is the same as in the double-pit VIP latrine but the two toilets are replaced by a single waterseal pan

**Fig. 6.14. Minimum distance between a pit and the external wall of a house**

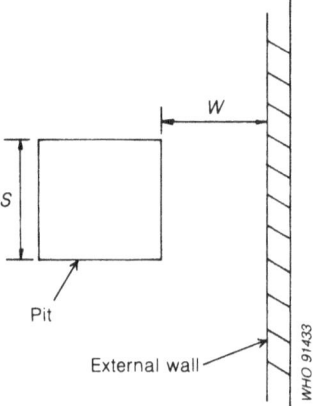

$W$ = depth of pit *or* 1.0 m provided $S$ is 1.0 m or less

**Fig. 6.15. Double-pit offset pour-flush latrine**

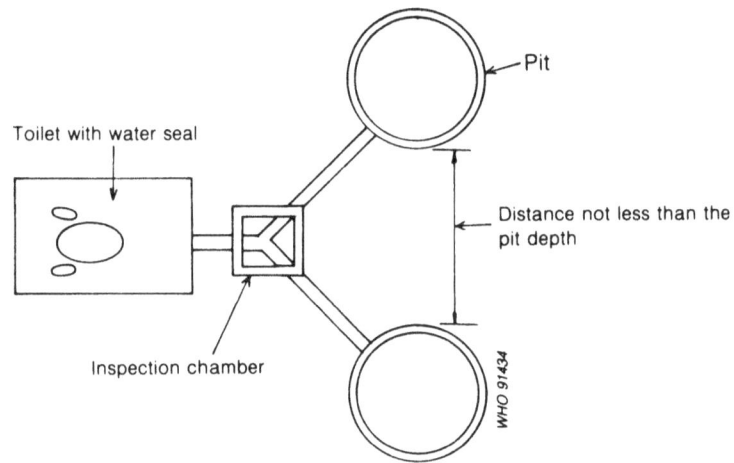

connected to both pits by pipes. An inspection chamber containing a Y junction is normally built between the pits and the pan so that the excreta can be channelled into either pit (Fig. 6.15).

Before a new latrine is brought into service, the inspection chamber is opened and one of the pipes leading to the pits is stopped off (a brick, stone, mound of clay or block of wood is quite satisfactory). The cover is then replaced and sealed to prevent gases escaping to the atmosphere. The latrine can now be used like an offset pour-flush toilet except that slightly more water may be required for flushing to prevent solids blocking the Y junction. Since one of the outlets from the chamber is blocked, all the contents of the toilet pan are directed into a

**Fig. 6.16. Some layout options for double-pit offset pour-flush latrines**

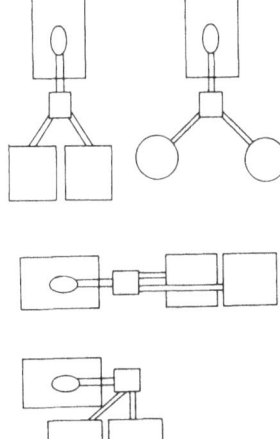

single pit. When the first pit is full, usually after a couple of years, the inspection chamber is opened and the stopper blocking the outlet pipe removed and placed in the other outlet pipe. The cover is again replaced and sealed. The pan contents now enter the second pit.

In a further two years the contents of the first pit will have decomposed and nearly all of the pathogenic organisms will have died. The lid of the first pit is taken off and the contents of the pit removed and disposed of or reused (see Annex 1). After replacing and sealing the lid, the first pit can be used again if the stopper in the Y junction is returned to its original position. In this way, the twin pits can be used indefinitely, each pit in turn being used for two years, rested for two years, emptied and then used again.

The positioning and shape of the pits is determined to a large extent by the space available. Some options are shown in Fig. 6.16. If possible, the distance between the pits should be not less than the depth of a pit. This is to reduce the possibility of liquid from the pit in use entering the pit not in use. If the pits have to be built adjacent to each other, the dividing wall should be non-porous. It can also be extended beyond the side-walls of the pit, to prevent cross-contamination. Alternatively, the pit lining can be constructed without holes for a distance of 300 mm either side of the dividing walls.

As with double-pit VIP latrines, double-pit pour-flush latrines are most useful in areas where it is not possible to dig a deep pit or where excreta are to be reused.

For proper operation it is most important that the construction, particularly of the Y junction, is carried out properly, and the user is made fully aware of how the latrine should be operated. Long-term support facilities to remind and assist the user in changing and emptying pits will greatly improve operational success.

## Raised pit latrines

Another way of dealing with the problem of difficult ground conditions close to the surface is to construct raised pit latrines. The pit is excavated as deep as possible, working at the end of the dry season in areas of high groundwater. The lining is extended above ground level until the desired pit volume is achieved.

If the pit extends more than 1.5 m below the ground there will probably be sufficient leaching area below ground for a pit latrine having a full depth of 3.5 m. In such cases, the lining above ground should be sealed by plastering both sides (Fig. 6.17). The minimum below-ground depth depends on the amount of water used in the pit and the permeability of the soil. Where insufficient infiltration area can be obtained below ground level, the raised portion of the pit can be surrounded by a mound of soil. The section of the lining above ground (excluding the top 0.5 m) can be used for infiltration provided the mound is made of permeable soil, well compacted with a stable side slope, and is thick enough to prevent filtrate seeping out of the sides

**Fig. 6.17 Raised pit latrine**

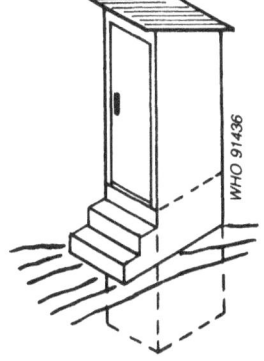

**Fig. 6.18. Mound latrine**

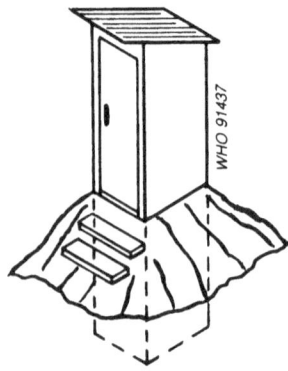

(Fig. 6.18). Earth mounds are not recommended on clay soils as the filtrate is likely to seep out at the base of the mound rather than infiltrate the ground.

Raised pits can be used in combination with any other type of pit latrine (VIP, pour-flush, double-pit). A common application is where the groundwater level is close to the surface. A slight raising of the pit may prevent splashing of the user or blockage of the pit inlet pipe by floating scum.

## Borehole latrines

Borehole latrines have an augered hole instead of a dug pit and may be sunk to a depth of 10 m or more, although a depth of 4–6 m is usual. Augered holes, 300–500 mm in diameter, may be dug quickly by hand or machine in areas where the soil is firm, stable and free from rocks or large stones. While a small diameter is easier to bore, the life of the pit is very short. For example a 300-mm hole 5 m deep will serve a family of five people for about two years.

The small diameter of the hole increases the likelihood of blockage, and the depth of the augered hole increases the danger of groundwater contamination. Even if the hole does not become blocked, the sides of the hole become soiled near the top, making fly infestation probable. However, borehole latrines are convenient for emergency or short-term use, because they can be prepared rapidly in great numbers, and light portable slabs may be used.

The holes should be lined for at least the top half-metre or so with an impervious material such as concrete or baked clay. Because of the small diameter and short life, the full depth is not usually lined.

## Septic tanks

Septic tanks are commonly used for wastewater treatment for individual households in low-density residential areas, for institutions such as schools and hospitals, and for small housing estates. The wastewater may be waste from toilets only, or may also include sullage.

The septic tank, in conjunction with its effluent disposal system, offers many of the advantages of conventional sewerage. However, septic tank systems are more expensive than most other on-site sanitation systems and are unlikely to be affordable by the poorer people in society. They also require sufficient piped water to flush all the wastes through the drains to the tanks.

### Treatment processes

Wastes from the toilet, and possibly kitchens and bathrooms, pass through drains into a sealed, watertight tank, where they are partially

**Fig. 6.19. Septic tank disposal system**

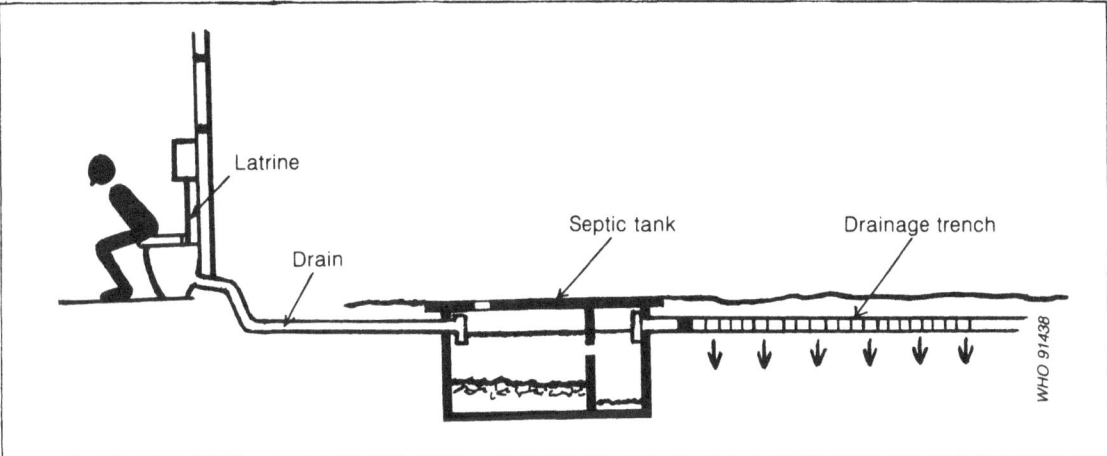

treated. After a period—usually 1–3 days—the partially treated liquid passes out of the tank and is disposed of, often to the ground through soakpits or tile drains in trenches (Fig. 6.19). Many of the problems with septic tank systems arise because inadequate consideration is given to the disposal of the tank effluent.

## Settlement

A principal aim of septic tank design is to achieve hydraulically quiescent conditions within the tank to assist the settlement by gravity of heavy solid particles. The settled material forms a layer of sludge on the bottom of the tank which must be removed periodically. The efficiency of removal of solids by settlement can be high. Majumder et al. (1960) reported removal of 80% of suspended solids in three tanks in West Bengal; similar removal rates were reported in a single tank near Bombay (Phadke et al., undated). However, much depends upon the retention time, the inlet and outlet arrangements, and the frequency of desludging. Large surges of flow entering the tank may cause a temporarily high concentration of suspended solids in the effluent owing to disturbance of the solids which have already settled out.

## Flotation

Grease, oil, and other materials that are less dense than water float up to the liquid surface, forming a layer of scum which can become quite hard. The liquid moves through the tank sandwiched between the scum and sludge.

### Sludge digestion and consolidation

Organic matter in the sludge and scum layers is broken down by anaerobic bacteria with a considerable amount of organic matter being converted into water and gases. Sludge at the bottom of the tank is consolidated owing to the weight of liquid and solids above. Hence the volume of sludge is considerably less than that of raw sewage solids entering the tank. Rising bubbles of gas cause a certain amount of disturbance to the liquid flow. The rate at which the digestion process proceeds increases with temperature, a maximum rate being achieved at about 35 °C. The use of ordinary household soap in normal amounts is unlikely to affect the digestion process (Truesdale & Mann, 1968). The use of abnormally large amounts of disinfectant causes bacteria to be killed off and thereby inhibits the digestion process.

### Stabilization of liquids

The liquid in the septic tank undergoes biochemical changes, but there are few data on the removal of pathogens. Both Majumder et al. (1960) and Phadke et al. (undated) found that although 80–90% of hookworm and *Ascaris* eggs were removed by the septic tanks studied, in absolute terms very large numbers of viable eggs were contained in the effluent, with 90% of effluent samples containing viable eggs.

Since the effluent from septic tanks is anaerobic and likely to contain large numbers of pathogens which can be a potential source of infection, it should not be used for crop irrigation nor should it be discharged to canals or surface-water drains without the permission of the local health authority.

## Design principles

The guiding principles in designing a septic tank are:

— to provide sufficient retention time for the sewage in the tank to allow separation of solids and stabilization of liquid;
— to provide stable quiescent hydraulic conditions for efficient settlement and flotation of solids;
— to ensure that the tank is large enough to store accumulated sludge and scum;
— to ensure that no blockages are likely to occur and that there is adequate ventilation of gases.

### Factors affecting design

The design method outlined below provides sufficient volume for both retention of liquid and storage of sludge and scum. The volume required for liquid retention depends upon the number of users, the amount of wastewater passed to the tank and whether sullage is accepted as well as waste from WCs. The volume for sludge and scum storage depends on the frequency with which the tank is desludged, the method of anal cleaning of the users and the temperature.

### Estimating the volume of a septic tank

#### Retention time

A sewage retention time of 24 hours is assumed to be sufficient. This should correspond to the situation immediately before the tank is desludged. After desludging the effective liquid retention time is greater because liquid then occupies the regions previously full of sludge and scum.

Codes of practice vary in their recommendations from a retention time of just less than 24 hours to about 72 hours. In theory, improved settlement results from a longer retention time, although the maximum rate of settlement is usually achieved within the first few hours. Settlement is impeded by flow disturbances caused by the inlet and outlet arrangements. The problem is likely to be greater in small tanks than large ones (whose hydraulic capacity is better able to damp out disturbances) and it is reasonable to assume that in large tanks correspondingly lower retention times can be used (Mara & Sinnatamby, 1986). The Brazilian code of practice (Associação Brasileira de Normas Técnicas, 1982) allows for reduced retention time in large tanks, such as those serving institutions or small communities. In summary, if the wastewater flowrate is $Q$ m³ per day, it recommends that the retention time should be $T$ hours, as follows:

If $Q$ is less than 6          $T = 24$
If $Q$ is between 6 and 14    $T = 33 - 1.5\,Q$
If $Q$ is greater than 14     $T = 12$

#### Liquid retention volume

If the septic tank accepts sullage as well as toilet waste, the sewage flow from a house or institution usually represents a high proportion of the water supplied. If the water supply per person is known, the sewage flow may be taken as 90% of the water supply. If the water supply exceeds about 250 litres per person per day, the excess is likely to be used for watering gardens. In most developing countries, the maximum sewage flow may be assumed to be between 100 and 200 litres per person per day.

If only WCs are connected to the septic tank, the sewage flow is estimated from an assumption about the number of times each user is likely to flush the WC. For example, each person may flush a 10-litre cistern four times a day.

The minimum capacity required for 24 hours' liquid retention is:

$$A = P \times q \text{ litres}$$

where   $A$ = required volume for 24 hours' liquid retention;
         $P$ = number of people served by the tank;
         $q$ = sewage flow per person (litres per person per day).

*Volume for sludge and scum storage*

The volume required for the accumulation of sludge and scum depends upon the factors discussed in Chapter 5. Pickford (1980) suggested the formula:

$$B = P \times N \times F \times S$$

where $B$ = the required sludge and scum storage capacity in litres;
       $N$ = the number of years between desludging (often 2–5 years; more frequent desludging may be assumed where there is a cheap and reliable emptying service);
       $F$ = a factor which relates the sludge digestion rate to temperature and the desludging interval, as shown in Table 6.2;
       $S$ = the rate of sludge and scum accumulation which may be taken as 25 litres per person per year for tanks receiving WC waste only, and 40 litres per person per year for tanks receiving WC waste and sullage.

**Table 6.2. Value of the sizing factor $F$ in determining volume for sludge and scum storage**

| Number of years between desludging | Value of $F$ | | |
|---|---|---|---|
| | Ambient temperature | | |
| | >20 °C throughout year | >10 °C throughout year | <10 °C during winter |
| 1 | 1.3 | 1.5 | 2.5 |
| 2 | 1.0 | 1.15 | 1.5 |
| 3 | 1.0 | 1.0 | 1.27 |
| 4 | 1.0 | 1.0 | 1.15 |
| 5 | 1.0 | 1.0 | 1.06 |
| 6 or more | 1.0 | 1.0 | 1.0 |

*Total tank volume*

The total capacity of the tank ($C$) is:

$$C = A + B \text{ litres}$$

In practice, there are limitations on the minimum size of tank that can be built; the guidelines described below are illustrated in the design examples given in Chapter 8.

*Shape and dimensions of septic tanks*

Having determined the overall capacity of the septic tank it is necessary to determine the depth, width and length. The aim is to achieve even distribution of flow so that there are no dead areas and no "short-circuiting" (that is, incoming flow shooting through the tank in less than the design retention time).

A tank may be divided into two or more compartments by baffle walls. Most settlement and digestion may occur in the first compartment with some suspended materials carried forward to the second. Surges of sewage entering the tank reduce the efficiency of settlement but have less effect in the second compartment. Laak (1980) reported a number of studies in which septic tanks with more than one compartment performed more effectively than single-compartment tanks. His survey also indicated that the first compartment should be twice as long as the second. Any advantage of more than two compartments has not been quantified.

The following guidelines can be used to determine the internal dimensions of a rectangular tank.

1. The depth of liquid from the tank floor to the outlet pipe invert should be not less than 1.2 m; a depth of at least 1.5 m is preferable. In addition a clear space of at least 300 mm should be left between the water level and the under-surface of the cover slab.
2. The width should be at least 600 mm as this is the minimum space in which a person can work when building or cleaning the tank. Some codes of practice recommend that the length should be 2 or 3 times the width.
3. For a tank of width $W$, the length of the first compartment should be $2W$ and the length of the second compartment should be $W$ (Fig. 6.20). In general, the depth should be not greater than the total length.

These guidelines give the minimum size of tank. There is no disadvantage in making a tank bigger than the minimum capacity. It may be cheaper to build larger tanks using whole blocks, rather than cutting blocks. Examples of septic tank design are given in Chapter 8.

**Fig. 6.20. Tank dimensions**

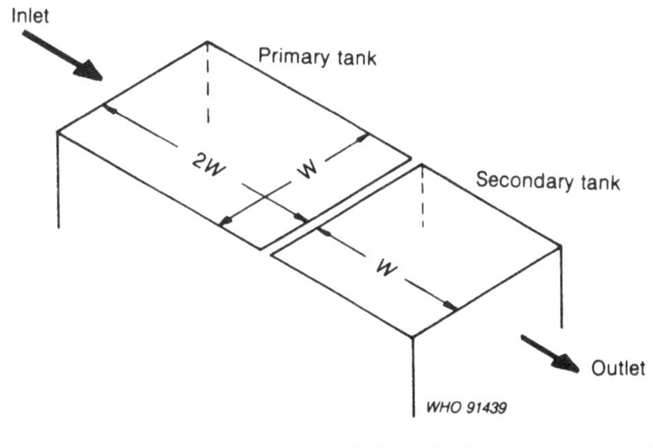

## Construction

The construction of a septic tank usually requires the assistance and supervision of an engineer or at least an experienced construction foreman. The design of the inlet and outlet is critical to the performance of the tank. Careful checking of levels is particularly important for large tanks that include complicated inlet, outlet and baffle-board arrangements.

For small household tanks, the floor is usually made of unreinforced concrete thick enough to withstand uplift pressure when the tank is empty. If the ground conditions are poor or the tank is large, the floor may have to be reinforced. The walls are commonly built of bricks, blocks or stone and should be rendered on the inside with cement mortar to make them watertight. Large reinforced concrete tanks serving groups of houses or institutions must be designed by a qualified engineer to ensure that they are structurally sound.

The tank cover or roof, which usually consists of one or more concrete slabs, must be strong enough to withstand any load that will be imposed.

Removable cover slabs should be provided over the inlet and outlet. Circular covers, rather than rectangular ones, have the advantage that they cannot fall into the tank when removed.

Septic tanks have been constructed from a variety of prefabricated sections, including large-diameter pipes. Experience has shown that the problems involved in fixing the inlet and outlet outweigh the advantages of using pipes. A number of proprietary designs of tank are manufactured from asbestos cement, glass-reinforced plastic and other materials and are sold commercially.

**Fig. 6.21. Septic tank inlet pipe**

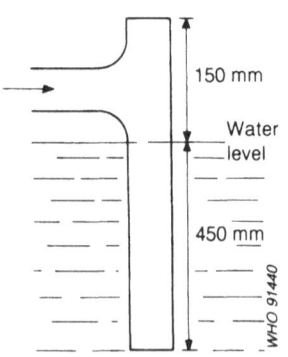

### Inlet

The sewage must enter the tank with the minimum possible disturbance to the liquid and solids already in the tank. Surges and turbulence reduce the efficiency of settlement and can cause large amounts of solid matter to be carried out in the tank effluent. Suitable inlet arrangements are shown in Fig. 6.21 and 6.24.

Surges are caused by flushing of the WC and emptying of sinks and baths. Their effect can be minimized by using drainpipes of not less than 100 mm in diameter and ensuring that the gradient of the pipe approaching the septic tank is flatter than about 1 in 66. Sizes and gradients of pipes between the building and the septic tank may be specified in local building regulations.

### Outlet

For septic tanks less than 1.2 m wide, a simple T-pipe arrangement can be used for the outlet. A removable cover above the T-pipe should be provided to permit clearance of any blockage. An alternative to the

**Fig. 6.22. Septic tank outlet baffle plate**

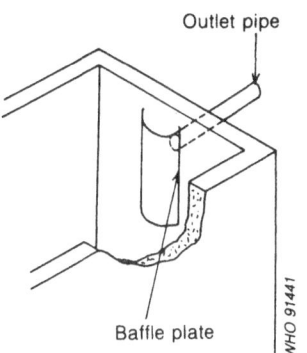

Outlet pipe

Baffle plate

WHO 91441

T-pipe is a baffle plate made of galvanized sheet, ferrocement or asbestos cement fitted round the outlet pipe (Fig. 6.22). A deflector may be provided below the outlet to reduce the possibility of settled sludge being resuspended and carried out of the tank. For tanks wider than 1.2 m, a full-width weir can be used to draw off the flow evenly across the tank. A scumboard should be fitted to prevent the scum washing over the weir (Fig. 6.23).

**Fig. 6.23. Septic tank outlet using full width weir**

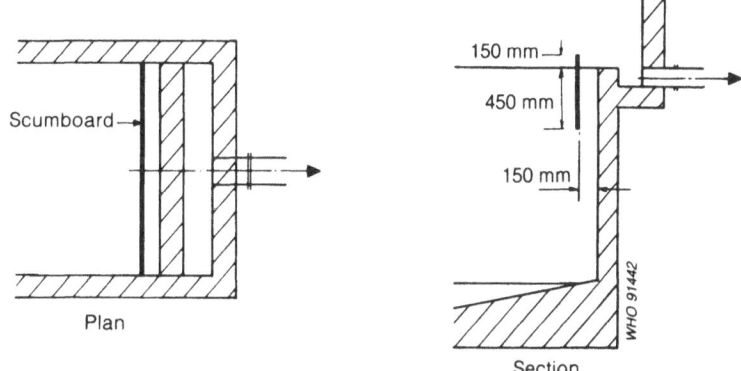

Scumboard

Plan

150 mm

450 mm

150 mm

WHO 91442

Section

## Dividing wall

If a tank is divided into two or more compartments, slots or a short length of pipe should be provided above the sludge level and below the scum level, as shown in Fig. 6.24. At least two should be installed to maintain uniform flow distribution across the tank.

## Ventilation of the tank

The anaerobic processes that occur in the tank produce gases which must be allowed a means of escape. If the drainage system of the house or other building has a ventilation pipe at the upper end, gases can escape from the septic tank along the drains. If the drainage system is not ventilated, a screened vent pipe should be provided from the septic tank itself.

## The tank floor

Some codes of practice recommend that the floor of a septic tank should slope downwards towards the inlet. There are two reasons: firstly, more sludge accumulates near the inlet, so a greater depth is desirable; secondly, the slope assists movement of sludge towards the inlet during desludging. For a two-compartment tank, the second compartment should have a horizontal floor and the first compartment

**Fig. 6.24. Septic tanks showing options for connections between compartments**

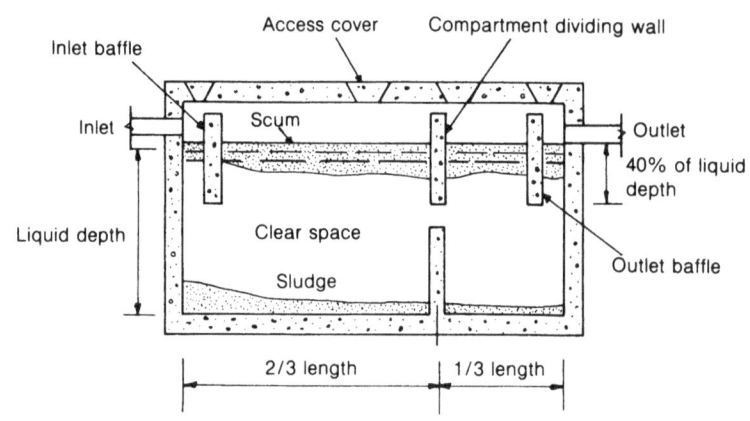

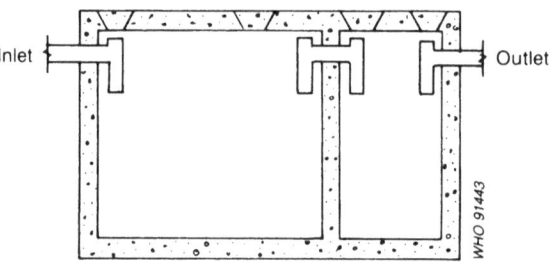

may slope at a gradient of 1 in 4 towards the inlet. When calculating the tank volume, it should be assumed that the floor is horizontal at the higher level. The effect of sloping the floor provides extra volume. The disadvantages of providing a sloping floor are that additional depth of excavation is required, the construction is made more complicated, and the cost of construction is increased.

## Operation and maintenance

### *Starting up the tank*

The process of anaerobic digestion of the sewage solids entering the tank can be slow in starting and it is a good idea to "seed" a new tank with sludge from a tank that has been operating for some time. This ensures that the necessary microorganisms are present in the tank to allow the digestion process to take place in a short time (McCarty, 1964).

### Maintenance

Routine inspection is necessary to check whether desludging is needed, and to ensure that there are no blockages at the inlet or outlet. A tank needs to be desludged when the sludge and scum occupy the volume specified in the design. A simple rule is to desludge when solids occupy between one-half and two-thirds of the total depth between the water level and the bottom of the tank. One of the difficulties with septic tanks is that they continue to operate even when the tank is almost full of solids. In this situation the inflow scours a channel through the sludge and may pass through the tank in a matter of minutes rather than remaining in the tank for the required retention time.

The most satisfactory method of sludge removal is by vacuum tanker. The sludge is pumped out of the tank through a flexible hose connected to a vacuum pump, which lifts the sludge into the tanker. If the bottom layers of sludge have cemented together they can be jetted with a water hose (which may be fitted to the tanker lorry) or broken up with a long-handled spade before being pumped out.

If a vacuum tanker is not available, the sludge must be bailed out manually using buckets. This is unpleasant work which exposes the operatives to health hazards.

Care must be taken to ensure that sludge is not spilled around the tank during emptying. Sludge removed from a septic tank includes fresh excreta and presents a risk of transmission of diseases of faecal origin. Careful disposal is therefore necessary.

When a septic tank is desludged it should not be fully washed out or disinfected. A small amount of sludge should be left in the tank to ensure continuing rapid digestion.

## Aqua-privies

An aqua-privy is a latrine set above or adjacent to a septic tank and is useful in situations in which there is a limited water supply (Fig. 6.25). Where the latrine is above the tank, a chute drop-pipe, 100–150 mm in diameter, hangs below the squat hole or latrine seat so that excreta drops directly into the tank below water level. The bottom of the pipe

**Fig. 6.25. Aqua-privy**

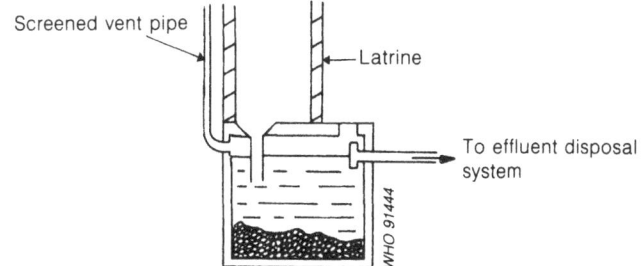

**Fig. 6.26. Aqua-privy with pan flushed by waste from a washing trough**

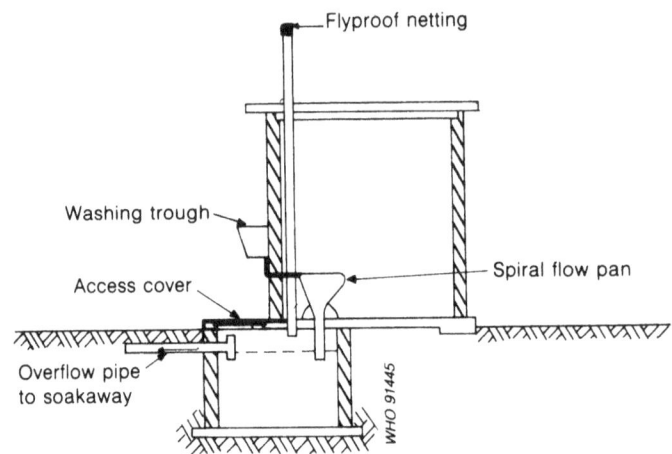

should be 75 mm below the liquid level in the tank, providing a seal which prevents gases escaping into the latrine superstructure and limits the access of flies and mosquitos to the tank. Alternatively the toilet may be fitted with a pan with a water seal. Where the latrine is adjacent to the tank, the pan with water seal is connected by a short pipe. Effluent from the tank goes to a soakpit, drainage trench or sewer. There is usually only a small flow of effluent and it is therefore very concentrated.

In order to keep a seal at the bottom of the drop-pipe it is essential that the water level in the tank is maintained. If the tank is completely watertight, a bucketful of water every day, used to clean the latrine, is sufficient to compensate for any losses due to evaporation. However, it has been found in practice that many tanks leak. In some places sullage is discharged into the tank (Fig. 6.26), but even this has not proved sufficient to ensure that the water level is above the bottom of the drop-pipe at all times. In Calcutta, aqua-privies used by people who use water for anal cleaning have a water seal incorporated in the drop-pipe below the pan (Pacey, 1978).

The design capacity of aqua-privy tanks may be calculated by the same procedure as for septic tanks. Regular removal of sludge and scum is essential, so a removable cover for desludging is required. A vent pipe is usually provided.

## Disposal of effluent from septic tanks and aqua-privies

A septic tank or aqua-privy is simply a combined retention tank and digester; apart from losses through seepage and evaporation, the outflow from the tank equals the inflow. The effluent is anaerobic and may contain a large number of pathogenic organisms. Although the removal of suspended solids can be high in percentage terms, the effluent is still concentrated in absolute terms, and the need for safe disposal of septic tank effluents cannot be too strongly stressed.

The effluent from large tanks dealing with sewage from groups of houses or from institutions may be treated by conventional sewage treatment processes such as percolating filters. Effluent from septic tanks and aqua-privies serving individual houses is normally discharged to soakpits or drainage trenches for infiltration into the ground. The infiltration capacities of the soil given in Table 5.4 (page 37) may be used to determine the required wall area of both soakpits and trenches.

Unfortunately it is not possible to predict the useful life of such disposal systems, which depend on the efficiency of the septic tank and the soil conditions. Pools of stagnant liquid often form when both toilet wastes and sullage are discharged to a septic tank and then to a drainage field which is too small or is clogged. This creates a potential health risk. Overloading of the drainage field may be avoided by allowing only toilet wastes to go to the septic tank. Sullage can be dealt with separately with fewer health risks than a mixture of partly treated toilet waste and sullage. Kalbermatten et al. (1980) proposed the use of a three-compartment septic tank, where sullage is introduced into the final compartment. It is suggested that the effluent infiltration rates may be double those for two-compartment tanks.

## Soakpits

Pits used to dispose of effluent from septic tanks are commonly 2–5 m deep with a diameter of 1.0–2.5 m. The capacity should be not less than that of the septic tank.

Depending on the nature of the soil and the local cost of stone and other building material, soakpits may either be lined or filled with stones or broken bricks. Linings are generally made of bricks, blocks or masonry with honeycomb construction or open joints (Fig. 6.27), as for the linings of pit latrines which are described in Chapter 7. The infiltration capacity of the soil may be increased by filling any space behind the lining with sand or gravel (Cairncross & Feachem, 1983). Hard material such as broken rock or broken kiln-dried bricks not less than 50 mm in diameter may be used to fill an unlined pit (Fig. 6.28).

Whether the main part of the pit is lined or filled, the top 500 mm should have a ring of blocks, bricks or masonry with full mortar joints to provide a firm support for the cover. The ring may be corbelled to reduce the size of the cover. Covers are usually made of reinforced concrete and may be buried by 200–300 mm of soil to keep out insects.

The area required for infiltration should be calculated from the data given in Chapter 5, as illustrated in Example 8.6 in Chapter 8. Increasing the diameter of the pit results in a disproportionate increase in the volume of excavation and in the cost of the cover slab compared with the increase of wall area. Therefore, if the required infiltration area is large, it may be more economical to provide drainage trenches.

**Fig. 6.27. Lined soakpit**

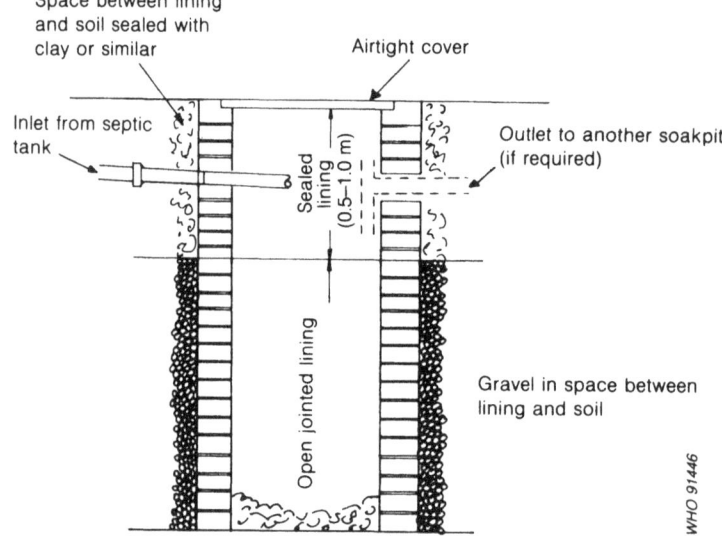

**Fig. 6.28. Unlined soakpit**

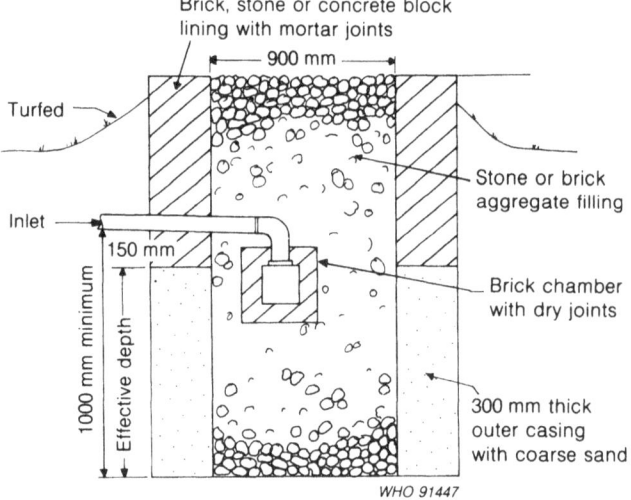

## Drainage trenches

The disposal of the large quantity of effluent from septic tanks is often effected in trenches which disperse the flow over a large area, reducing the risk of overloading at one place. The trenches make up a drainage field. The effluent is carried in pipes which are normally 100 mm in diameter with a gap of about 10 mm between each pipe. Unglazed stoneware pipes (tile drains) are often used, either with plain ends or with spigot and socket joints. The upper part of the gap between plain-end pipes may be covered with strips of tarred paper or plastic sheet to prevent entry of sand or silt. With spigot and socket pipes, a small stone or cement fillet can be placed on each socket to centre the adjoining spigot (Fig. 6.29).

Drainage trenches are usually dug with a width of 300–500 mm and a depth of 600–1000 mm below the top of the pipes. A common practice is to lay the pipes at a gradient of 0.2–0.3% on a bed of gravel, the stones with a diameter of 20–50 mm. Soil is returned to a depth of 300–500 mm above the stones, with a barrier of straw or building paper to prevent soil washing down (Fig. 6.30).

If more than one trench is needed it is recommended that the drains be laid in series (Cotteral & Norris, 1969). Drains in series are either full or empty, allowing the soil alongside empty drains to recover under aerobic conditions (Fig. 6.31). If drains are laid in parallel, there is a

**Fig. 6.29. Open pipe joint in a drainage trench**

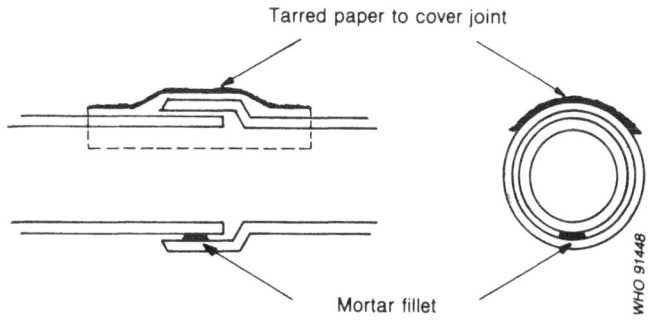

**Fig. 6.30. Drainage trench**

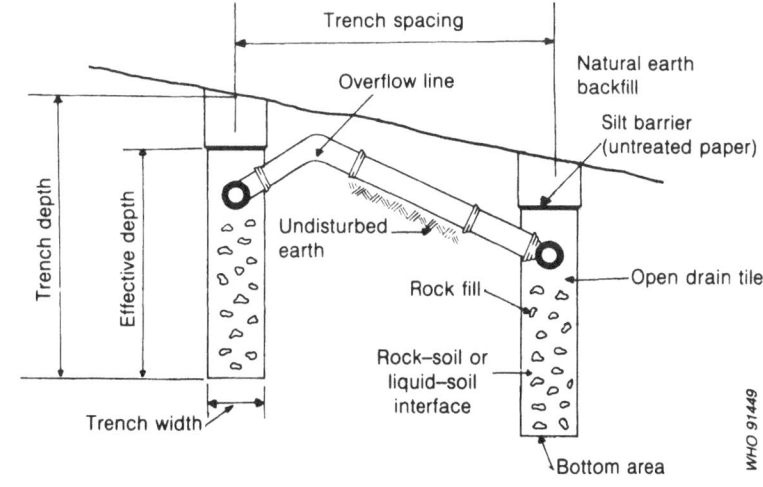

**Fig. 6.31. Drainage trenches laid in series in a drainage field. A–A indicates section shown in Fig. 6.30**

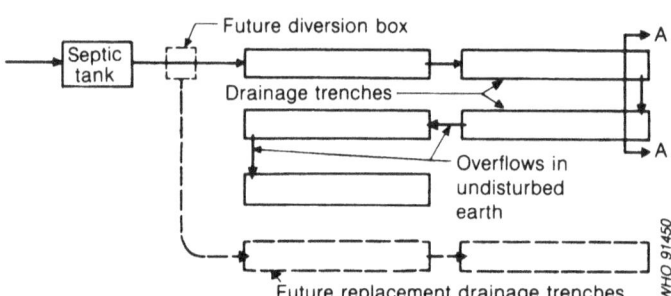

tendency for all trenches to contain some effluent. Trenches should be 2 m apart, or twice the trench depth if this is greater than 1 m.

The length of trench should be calculated by dividing the flow of effluent by the infiltration rate, allowing for the area of both sides of the trench, as illustrated by the examples given in Chapter 8.

## Composting latrines

The value of composting excreta with dry organic matter is discussed in Annex 1. Composting toilets are of two types: those such as double-vault latrines, which use anaerobic bacteria, and continuous composting latrines, which make use of aerobic bacteria.

### Double-vault latrines

Each latrine consists of two chambers or vaults used alternately (Fig. 6.32). Initially a layer of about 100 mm of absorbent organic material such as dry earth is put in the bottom of one vault, which is then used for defecation. After each use, the faeces are covered with wood ash or similar material to deodorize the decomposing faeces and soak up excess moisture.

When the vault is three-quarters full, the contents are levelled with a stick and the vault is completely filled with dry powdered earth. The squat hole is then sealed. While the contents of the first vault are decomposing anaerobically, the second vault is used. When the second tank is full, the first one is emptied through a door near the bottom and the chamber is reused. The contents may be used as a soil conditioner.

Each vault should be large enough to hold at least two years' accumulation of wastes so that most pathogenic organisms die off before the compost is removed. Recommended vault sizes range from 1.1 m³ (Winblad & Kalama, 1985) to 2.23 m³ (Wagner & Lanoix, 1958).

Normally the superstructure is built over both vaults, with a squat hole over each vault. A cover sealed with lime mortar or clay should be

**Fig. 6.32. Double-vault latrine**

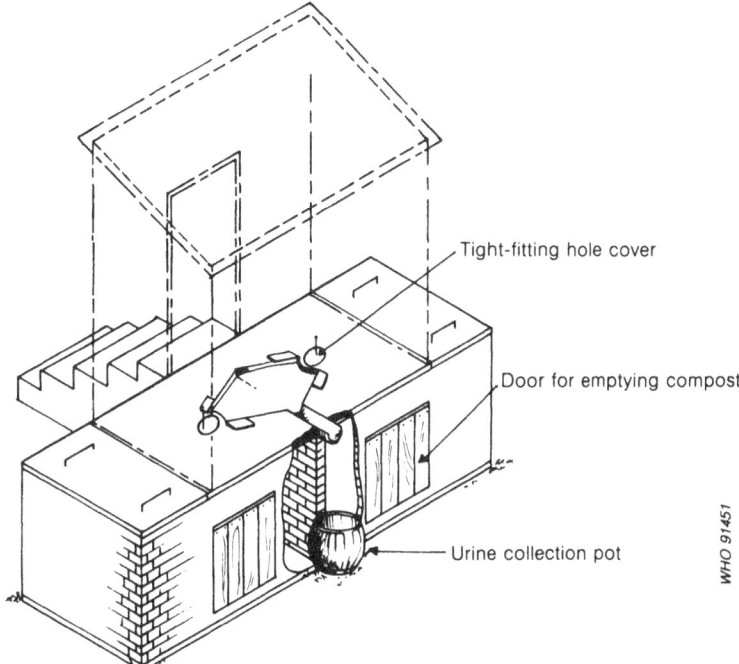

Tight-fitting hole cover

Door for emptying compost

Urine collection pot

WHO 91451

fitted in the squat hole above the chamber not in use. A flyproof lid should be placed on the other hole when it is not being used for defecation. Flyproof vent pipes may be provided to avoid odour nuisance in the latrine, although covering the faeces with ash is reported to be sufficient to eliminate bad smells.

Control of the moisture content is vital for proper operation of the latrine. Consequently composting latrines are not appropriate where water is used for anal cleaning. It is usual to collect urine separately, dilute it with 3–6 parts of water and use it as a fertilizer (although this may cause a health hazard). Some latrines are constructed with soakpits below the vaults so that excess moisture can drain into the ground (Fig. 6.33). This allows for the disposal of urine into the vaults but with consequent loss of a valuable fertilizer and possible pollution of the groundwater. Wood ash, straw, sawdust, grass cuttings, vegetable wastes and other organic material must be put into vaults to control moisture content and improve the quality of the final compost.

Besides providing a reusable resource, the double-vault latrine has the added advantage that it can be built anywhere. Since the vault contents are kept dry, there is no pollution of the surrounding ground, even if the vault is buried. In rocky areas or where the water table is high the vaults may be built above ground. Walls and base should be watertight.

**Fig. 6.33. Double-vault latrine with soakpits**

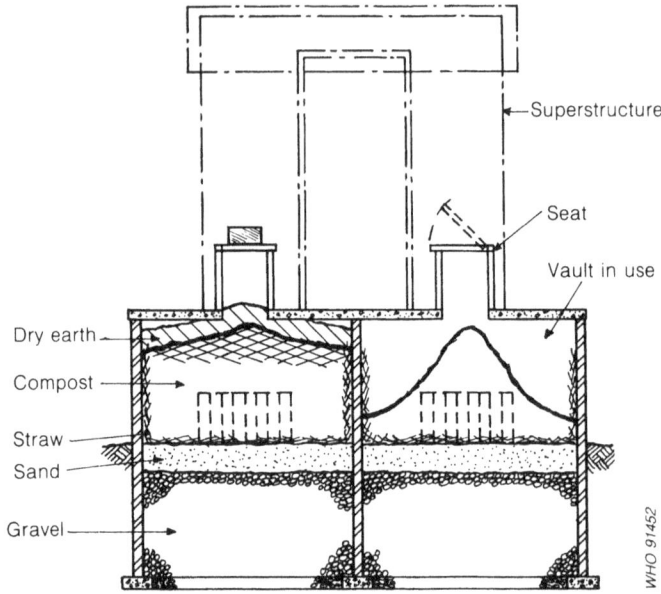

Double-vault composting latrines have been successfully used in Viet Nam (McMichael, 1976) and Guatemala (Buren et al., 1984). When tried elsewhere they have usually been unsatisfactory. Most of the disadvantages revolve round the problem of controlling the moisture content. Proper operation of the latrine is difficult to understand and considerable effort may be required to educate local people in its use. The contents are often allowed to become too wet, making the vault difficult to empty and malodorous.

## Continuous composting toilets

These consist of watertight sloping chambers about 3 m in length. Excreta fall into the chamber from a toilet. Dry organic kitchen and garden waste is tipped in through a separate opening (Fig. 6.34).

Inverted U-shaped ducts and a ventilation pipe encourage the passage of air through the mass, preventing it from becoming anaerobic and allowing excess moisture to evaporate. As new material enters at the top of the chamber, older material gradually moves to the bottom and then slides into a smaller compartment from which it is removed periodically.

Such toilets have proved satisfactory in holiday homes and other isolated buildings in industrialized countries, where they are sometimes installed in a cellar beneath the latrine and kitchen.

Attempts have been made in Botswana and the United Republic of Tanzania to adapt the design to suit African materials and customs (Winblad & Kalama, 1985) using tanks made with concrete or sand and

**Fig. 6.34. Continuous composting toilet**

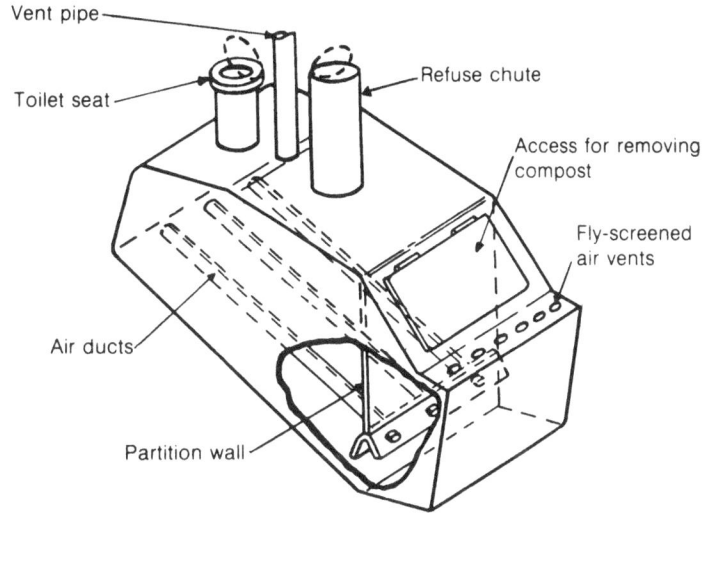

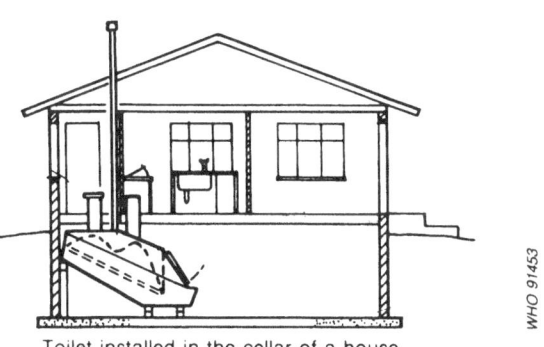

Toilet installed in the cellar of a house

cement blocks. They were found to be inappropriate because of their high cost and sensitivity to user operation. Retaining the proper carbon–nitrogen balance and moisture content is crucial to proper operation. In practice, it has been found that moisture content is the most difficult to control. Fly and odour problems are also common, particularly soon after commissioning.

## Multiple latrines

In some cultures there is a preference for separate latrines for men and women or adults and children. There is also a need for multiple latrines at places where large numbers of people meet, such as schools, restaurants, offices, etc.

Latrines fitted with a water seal may be connected to a common pit by drains (Fig. 6.35). VIP latrines may also be constructed over a common pit but the number of toilet holes using a single vent pipe should be limited to two. A multiple double-pit VIP latrine has been developed where each cubicle has two holes or seats (Fig. 6.36). These holes are used alternately in the same way as double-pit VIPs. The holes are used in such a way that the two holes which serve a pit are in use (or not in use) at the same time. The holes not being used are sealed. The dividing walls in the pit must extend to the full height of the pit.

**Fig. 6.35. Connecting a number of pour-flush latrines to a common pit**

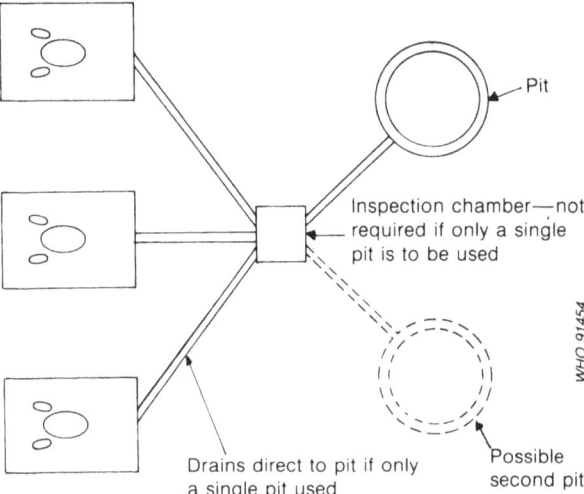

## Other latrines

### Bucket latrines

The system in which excreta are removed from bucket latrines (also called nightsoil latrines or earth closets) is one of the oldest forms of organized sanitation. Bucket latrines are still found in many towns and cities in Africa, Latin America and Asia, because their low capital cost makes them attractive to underfunded local authorities.

In some rural and periurban areas, members of households take nightsoil to manure heaps or apply it directly to fields as fertilizer. In towns and cities, nightsoil is often collected by sweepers engaged by householders on contract, or by the local authorities. Buckets are usually emptied into larger containers near the latrine. In some places labourers carry these containers by hand or on their heads; hand-carts, animal-drawn carts, bicycles and tricycles are also used.

**Fig. 6.36. Multiple double-pit VIP latrine**

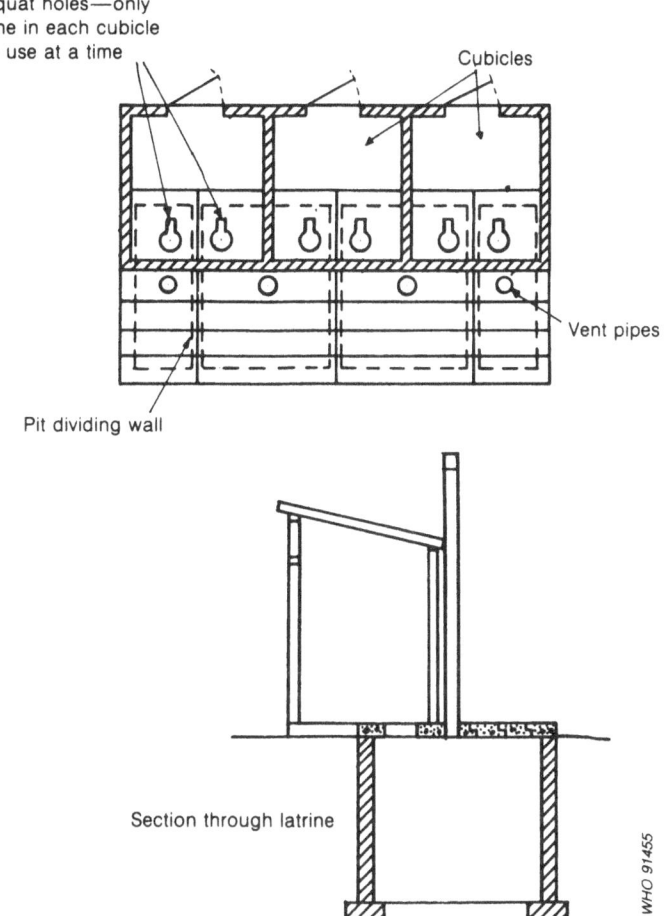

For the reasons given in Chapter 4, nightsoil collection should never be considered as an option for sanitation improvement programmes, and all existing bucket latrines should be replaced as soon as possible.

The number of bucket latrines is declining rapidly. However, for many years to come, some people will have to rely on bucket latrines as their only form of sanitation. The following paragraphs give suggestions for improvements to existing systems until they can be replaced by more acceptable forms of sanitation.

### Good operation

A container made of non-corrosive material is placed beneath a squatting slab or seat in the bucket chamber, with rear doors which should be kept shut except during removal and replacement of the bucket.

The bucket chamber should be cleaned whenever the bucket is removed. The squat hole should be covered by a flyproof cover when not in use. The cover of the seat should be hinged (Fig. 6.37) and the cover of the squatting slab should have a long handle.

At regular intervals (preferably each night) the container should be removed and replaced by a clean one. Full containers should be taken to depots or transfer stations where they are emptied, washed and disinfected with a phenol or cresol type of disinfectant. In some towns it is the practice to provide two buckets painted in different colours for each latrine. Containers should be kept covered with tight-fitting lids while in transit and the operators should be provided with full protective clothing. Proper supervision and management are essential. Defective buckets should be repaired or replaced and transport vehicles should be kept in good order.

In some systems, urine is diverted away from the buckets to reduce the volume to be dealt with. It is usually channelled to soakpits, but may be collected separately and used directly as fertilizer. Water used for washing latrines and bucket-chambers should pass to soakpits, and should not be allowed to pollute the ground around the latrines.

## Disposal methods

The practice of dumping nightsoil indiscriminately into streams or on open land is objectionable and causes health hazards.

**Fig. 6.37. Bucket latrine**

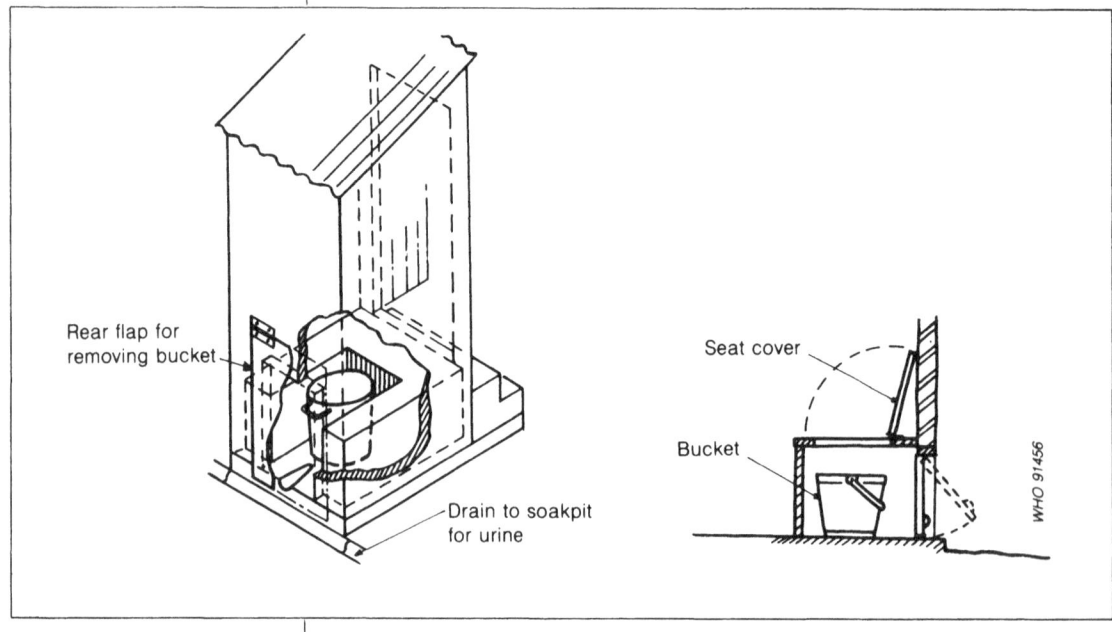

Rear flap for removing bucket

Drain to soakpit for urine

Seat cover

Bucket

WHO 91456

*Sewers*

Bucket latrines are sometimes found in towns that are partially provided with sewers, in which case it may be convenient to discharge the nightsoil into a main sewer. Tipping points on sewers require careful design to prevent contamination of surrounding areas and should be as near to the sewage works as possible. Extra water may have to be added to prevent blockage of the sewers.

*Sewage treatment works*

Nightsoil may be discharged into the sewage flow at the works inlet, at sedimentation or aeration tanks, or directly to waste stabilization ponds or sludge digestion tanks.

*Trenching*

Trenches about 1 m deep and 1 m wide may be filled with nightsoil to within not less than 300 mm of the top. The trench is then backfilled with excavated soil, which should be well compacted to prevent the emergence of flies or the excreta being dug up by animals (Fig. 6.38). At the end of each day any exposed excreta must be covered with at least 200 mm of soil, well compacted. After backfilling, the trench should remain untouched for at least two years, after which it can be re-excavated for reuse and the contents used as fertilizer. The trenching site should be close to the collection area but away from residential areas. It should have deep and porous soil, be well above the water table, and not be subject to flooding.

*Reuse*

Nightsoil can be used as a fertilizer after all pathogens have been destroyed. It may also be added to ponds for fish cultivation (see Annex 1).

**Fig. 6.38. Disposing of excreta from bucket latrines by trenching**

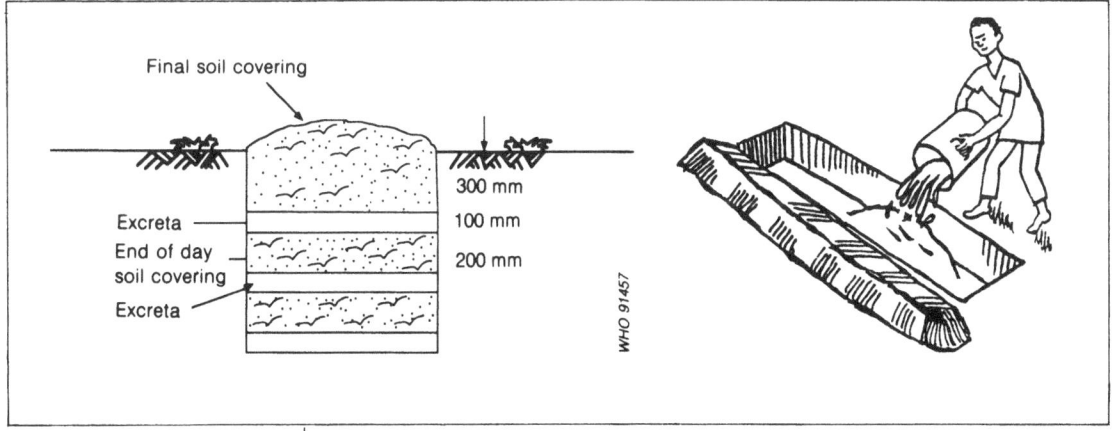

## Vault latrines

Vault latrines are a way of overcoming the problem of frequent emptying needed with bucket latrine systems. A watertight tank or vault below or close to a latrine is used to collect faeces, urine and sometimes sullage. The capacity of the vault is often sufficient for 2–3 weeks' accumulation of excreta, after which time the vault is emptied. The system is satisfactory if collection is reliable and hygienic, and the vaults are properly flyproofed, vented and fitted with water-seal toilets.

In some places, the contents of vaults are bailed out by hand and taken away in tanks mounted on carts. This is highly undesirable. Trials with manually operated pumps to empty vault contents have not been very successful because with a low pumping rate (about 400 litres per hour) complete evacuation of the vault is a long and tedious operation. This method is obviously also undesirable.

Motorized vacuum tankers can provide safe removal but must be backed up by good institutional support for operation and maintenance. Most vacuum tankers cannot lift vault contents if the proportion of solids exceeds about 12%, but some have facilities for adding water to vaults before lifting the contents.

Sufficient extra space to allow for irregularities in collection time should be planned for in designing vault capacity. In communities where finance, spare parts and good maintenance are available, the additional space needed may be only 15–20%. However, where vehicle maintenance is poor, an allowance of 50% may be advisable.

The performance of vaults has been mixed, mainly dependent on the levels of finance and vehicle maintenance. Poorly constructed vaults are common, leading to problems with odour and flies, ground pollution and thickening of the vault contents. It is not recommended that new vault latrines be constructed.

## Cesspits

Cesspits, like vaults, are watertight tanks with sealed covers (to keep out mosquitos). They differ from vaults in that they are usually located outside the premises and collect sullage as well as the wastes from water closets. The capacity may be sufficient for up to several months' use (Fig. 6.39). The cost of providing a regular removal service for all the wastewater from a house with a good supply of piped water can be very high, making cesspits an expensive form of sanitation.

## Chemical toilets

Modern chemical toilets are normally of the following types:

- a cylindrical bucket fitted with a plastic seat and lid; the capacity is usually 20–30 litres; after the bucket has been emptied and cleaned, about 50 mm depth of fluid is put in;

**Fig. 6.39. Cesspit**

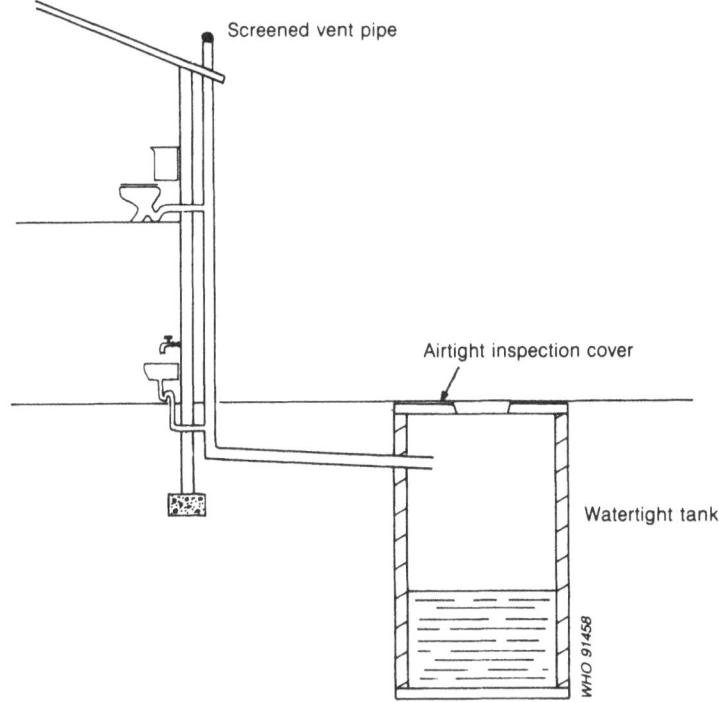

**Fig. 6.40. Manually flushed chemical toilet**

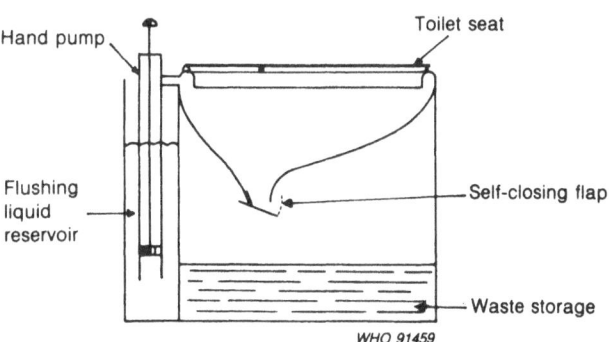

- two tanks: the flushing-liquid reservoir contains a mixture of fresh water and a deodorizing chemical which is pumped manually to the rim of the pan; discharge is to the waste-storage tank (Fig. 6.40);
- a single tank in which a flushing pan is fitted; a manual or electrically operated pump recirculates oil, drawing it from the base of the tank through a filter and discharging it around the rim of the pan; the

**Fig. 6.41. Recirculating oil toilet**

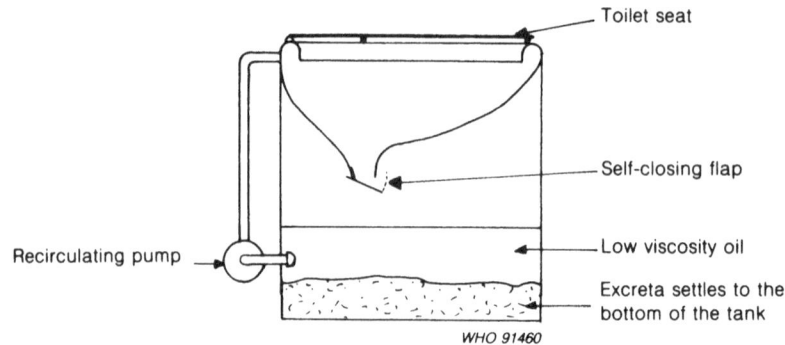

pan has a counter-balanced flap so that the contents cannot be seen (Fig. 6.41).

The fluid is normally a chemical diluted with water which renders excreta harmless and odourless. When containers are full, the contents are tipped into pits or sewers, or pumped into storage tanks.

Chemical toilets are used in aircraft, long-distance coaches, caravans, vacation homes and construction sites. The chemical is expensive.

## Overhung latrines

An overhung latrine consists of a superstructure and floor built over water (Fig. 6.42). A squat hole in the floor allows excreta to fall into the water. A chute is sometimes provided from the floor to the water. Overhung latrines should never be built in places where pit latrines can be provided. However, they may be the only possible form of sanitation for people living on land that is continuously or seasonally covered with water.

Wagner & Lanoix (1958) suggested that such latrines might be acceptable provided the following conditions are met.

- The receiving water is of sufficient salinity all year round to prevent human consumption.
- The latrine is installed over water that is sufficiently deep to ensure that the bed is never exposed during low tide or the dry season.
- Every effort is made to select a site from where floating solids will be carried away from the village.
- The walkways, piers, squatting openings, and superstructures are made structurally safe for adults and children.
- The excreta are not deposited in still water or into water that will be used for recreation.

**Fig. 6.42. Overhung latrine**

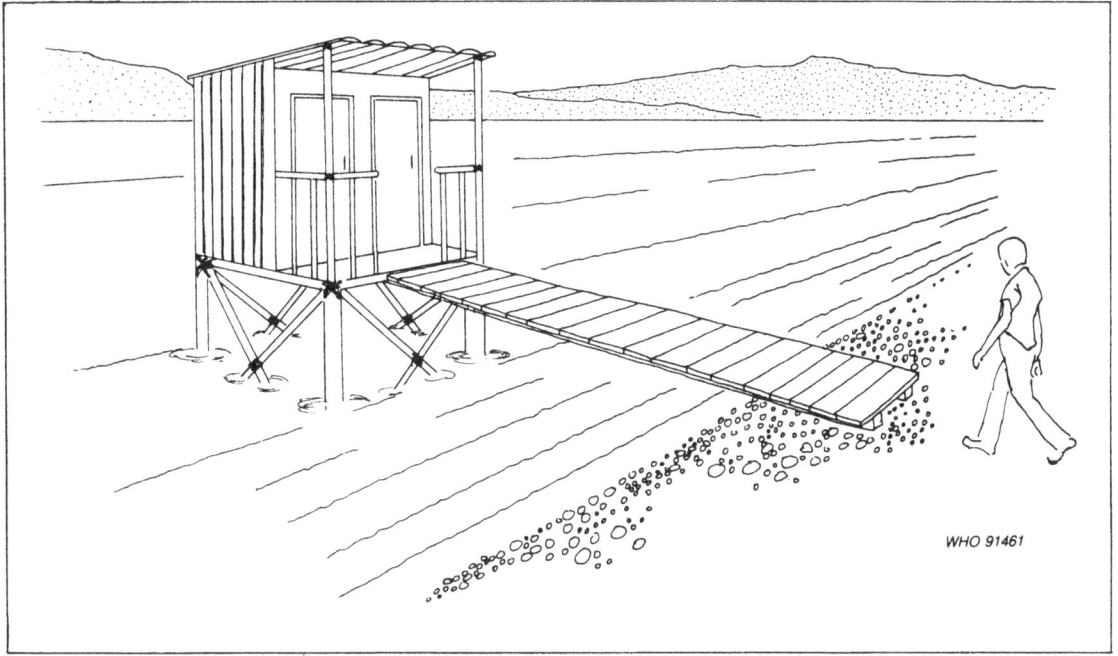

WHO 91461

CHAPTER 7
# Components and construction of latrines

Many components of sanitation systems are common to different types of latrines. In this chapter, the technical details of the following components are considered:

— pits and pit linings;
— latrine floors, which may be cast directly on the ground where the pit or vault is offset;
— slabs, supported over direct or offset pits;
— footrests and squat holes;
— seats;
— water seals, pans, pipes and junction chambers;
— vent pipes;
— superstructures.

## Pits

### Excavation

Most pit latrines provide sanitation for a single household, usually necessitating a pit about 1 m across and 3 m or more in depth (although much larger pits are common in some areas), or two shallow pits of up to 1.5 m in depth. The pit may be circular, square or rectangular in plan. Circular pits are more stable because of the natural arching effect of the ground around the hole, with no sharp corners to concentrate the stresses (Fig. 7.1). However, people often find that square or rectangular pits are easier to dig. The depth of the pits often follows local traditions. It is usually advantageous to dig the pit as deep as possible, but this depends on soil conditions, cost of lining and the level of the groundwater.

### Pit linings

The need for a pit lining depends upon the type of latrine under construction and the condition of the soil. In septic tanks and aqua-privies, for example, which require watertight compartments, the pit is always lined. However, in pit latrines it is only necessary to have a lining if the soil is likely to collapse during the life span of the latrine.

It is not easy to decide in advance whether a soil will be self-supporting. If other excavations in the locality (such as shallow wells) have proved to be self-supporting over a number of years, then it is

**Fig. 7.1. Strength of different pit shapes**

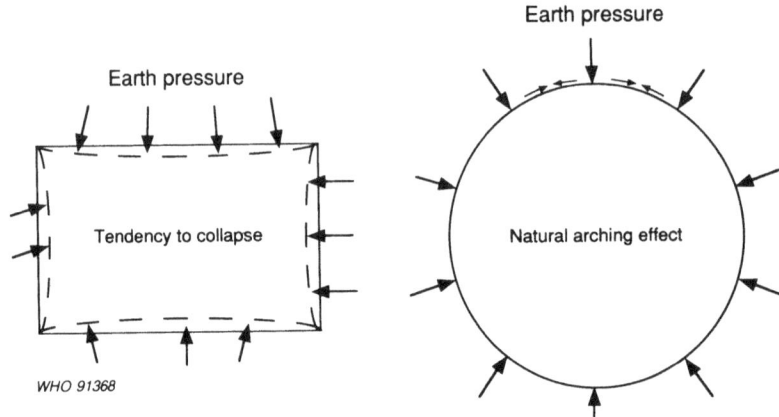

probably safe to assume that a pit for a latrine can be dug without support. Granular soils such as sands and gravels normally require support. Cohesive soils, such as silts and clays, and soils with a high proportion of iron oxides, such as laterites, are often self-supporting. However, silts and clays may lose their self-supporting properties when wet, particularly where there is a varying water table.

If there is any doubt about the conditions it is better to assume that the soil is not self-supporting. Increasingly it is recommended that all pits should be lined, especially where the design life is over five years. Failure of an unlined deep pit can be extremely hazardous for the person excavating it. If the failure occurs some years later it can be expensive for the owner and disturbing for the users. In all cases the top 300–500 mm should be lined and sealed to support the slab (and where necessary the superstructure) and to prevent contamination of the surface and entry of vermin.

The lining may be of any material that supports the soil and that will last as long as the design life of the pit. Commonly, materials such as fired bricks, concrete blocks, concrete, ferrocement and local stone are used, but stabilized soil blocks, old oil drums (though with a limited life in corrosive groundwater) and unglazed fired clay pipes have also been successful.

Quarried stone, where available cheaply, makes a satisfactory lining. The more regular blocks should be used for the top 500 mm with mortar joints. Less-regular stone can be used for the remainder of the lining without mortar in the vertical joints. The builders or masons must be skilled and experienced if the lining is to last a reasonable length of time. Where local stone is used, its durability must be confirmed. Some stone will deteriorate when exposed to air or water or to frequent changes between wet and dry conditions.

The use of timber or bamboo is not generally recommended, since they are subject to insect and fungal attack and often have a limited life.

Some hard woods can be satisfactory provided they are treated with tar, creosote or other preservative to lengthen their life. Care must be taken to ensure that none of the preservatives leach into the ground-water as even low levels of some preservatives can be toxic (WHO, 1984). Woven cane and bamboo have been used for the lower part of a lining with stronger materials used for the top 500 mm. However, unless the pits are designed to have an extremely short life, cane and bamboo should be avoided.

## Construction

### *Shallow pits*

In almost all cases, pits of up to 1.5 m in depth can be excavated to their full depth and then lined from the bottom up. If the soil is very loose, the sides of the excavation may have to be sloped to prevent collapse. The space between the lining and the soil can then be backfilled, preferably with a granular material such as sand or gravel. Granular materials are used because they fill the space between the soil and the lining without leaving large voids. They also act as a filter to prevent soil particles being washed into the pit. Voids behind the lining produce locally increased loads on the lining which may cause collapse.

It is usual to provide a foundation for the lining similar to that provided for a domestic house. In most soils, a foundation width equal to twice the wall thickness is usually sufficient (Fig. 7.2). In very soft ground it may be necessary to construct wider foundations to prevent the weight of the lining itself forcing it into the soil (Fig. 7.3). Where the superstructure load is not directly applied to the lining, a widened foundation may not be required since the load applied to the ground at the base of the lining is small and considerable skin friction builds up between the sides of the lining and the ground.

Soakpits or leaching pits require a porous lining to allow the wastewater to escape into the ground. The method of achieving this depends upon the lining material used. With bricks, blocks or local

**Fig. 7.2. Lining for a shallow pit in firm ground**

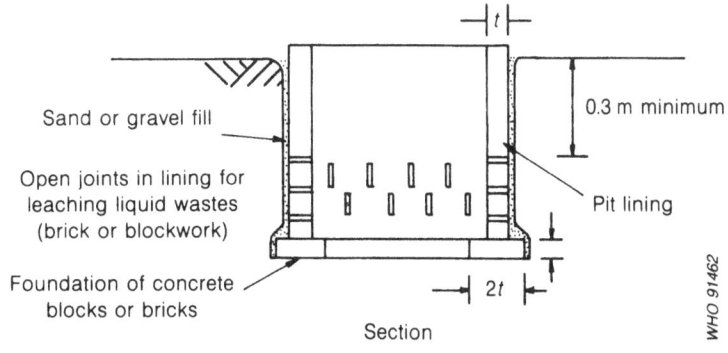

Sand or gravel fill

Open joints in lining for leaching liquid wastes (brick or blockwork)

Foundation of concrete blocks or bricks

0.3 m minimum

Pit lining

$t$

$2t$

Section

WHO 91462

87

**Fig. 7.3. Lining for a shallow pit in soft ground**

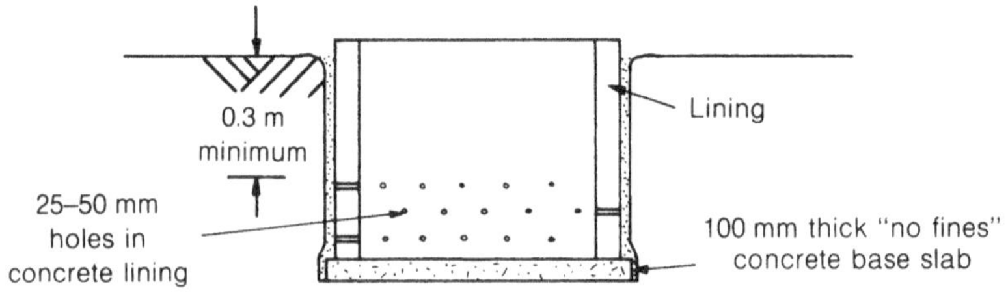

0.3 m
minimum

Lining

25–50 mm
holes in
concrete lining

100 mm thick "no fines"
concrete base slab

Section

WHO 91463

stone, a proportion of the vertical joints are left unmortared. These unmortared joints may be confined to specific courses (e.g., every third or fourth course) rather than being spread throughout the lining. This enables the fully mortared courses to carry the load exerted by the soil on the lining. Where the ground is relatively strong, a more open, honeycomb technique is used, with only small dabs of mortar joining the masonry. Alternatively, specially manufactured bricks with angled ends to suit round pits and a central opening to allow for infiltration may be used (D. J. T. Webb, personal communication).

Concrete, ferrocement and fired clay ring linings are made porous by creating holes of 25–50 mm in diameter through the lining. Alternatively, the ring joints are held open by small stones or bricks. Additionally, concrete linings may be made of "no fines" concrete, that is, concrete without any fine aggregate (sand). A mix of one part of cement to four parts of clean gravel (with stones of 6–18 mm in diameter) is suitable. Where precast rings are used, the upper and lower 100 mm of the ring should be made of conventional concrete for extra strength.

## Deep pits

The method of excavating deep pits depends upon the stability of the soil during the construction period. In soils that are self-supporting, the pit may be dug to its full depth and the lining installed afterwards. If the ground is not self-supporting, the lining must be constructed as the pit is dug.

Where a lining is not required for support during excavation, the pit is dug to the full depth, making allowance for the thickness of the lining to be installed subsequently. Accurate dimensions are maintained by using a plumb bob to ensure verticality and a template, either circular or rectangular to retain the horizontal dimensions. Ensuring correct dimensions minimizes the costs of lining and backfilling. Sometimes the soil near the surface is weathered and likely to collapse. In that case, the top metre of soil may be supported with a temporary lining (Fig. 7.4). If the finished lining is to be of precast concrete rings, then

**Fig. 7.4. Excavation for a pit to be lined with precast concrete rings**

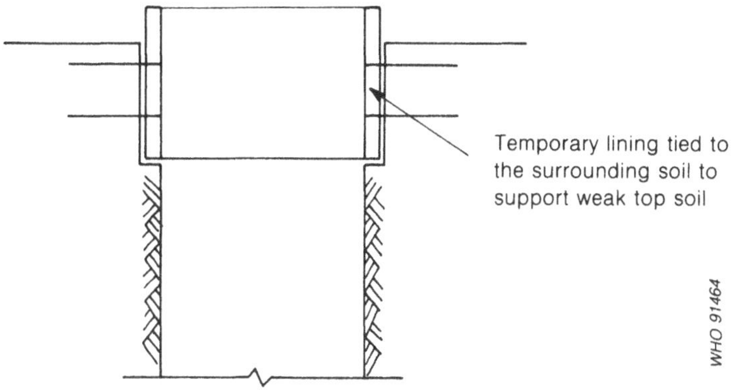

Temporary lining tied to
the surrounding soil to
support weak top soil

WHO 91464

the top metre of soil will have to be excavated to a larger diameter so that the rings can pass inside the temporary lining.

When the hole has been excavated to the design depth, the bottom is levelled and cleaned. In firm ground, a foundation can be constructed by cutting a groove into the walls of the pit and building a ring beam. In exceptionally soft ground, where the lining is likely to sink into the floor of the pit, the ring beam foundation can be replaced by a floor slab of "no fines" concrete, 75–100 mm in thickness, covering the whole base of the pit. This will distribute the weight of the lining over a larger area of the pit base, thus reducing the load per unit area and preventing upwards heave of the soil (see Fig. 7.3).

### Construction of linings

#### Precast rings
The use of precast concrete (Fig. 7.5) or fired clay rings for the lining of pits has the advantage that the lining can be prepared before excavation begins. This is particularly useful in weaker soils because it reduces the time the soil remains unsupported. The rings to be placed at the bottom of the hole may be porous, designed to allow the liquid wastes to seep into the surrounding soils or they may be sealed to create a wet tank, designed to increase the rate of sludge digestion. The ring nearest to the surface should be fully sealed to prevent entry of surface water and rodents and also contamination of the soil. As with shallow pits, any space between the back of the rings and the soil should be filled with sand or gravel.

#### Brick, blockwork and stone lining
These are built in a similar way to precast concrete linings, i.e., by building up from the foundations. With very deep pits it may be wise to allow time for the cement mortar to gain strength before filling any space behind the lining, to prevent the weight of the fill from deforming

**Fig. 7.5. Pit bottom lined with precast concrete rings**

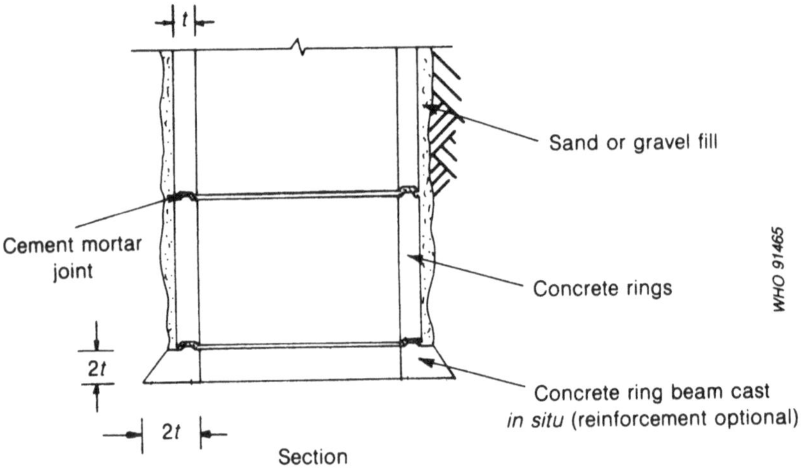

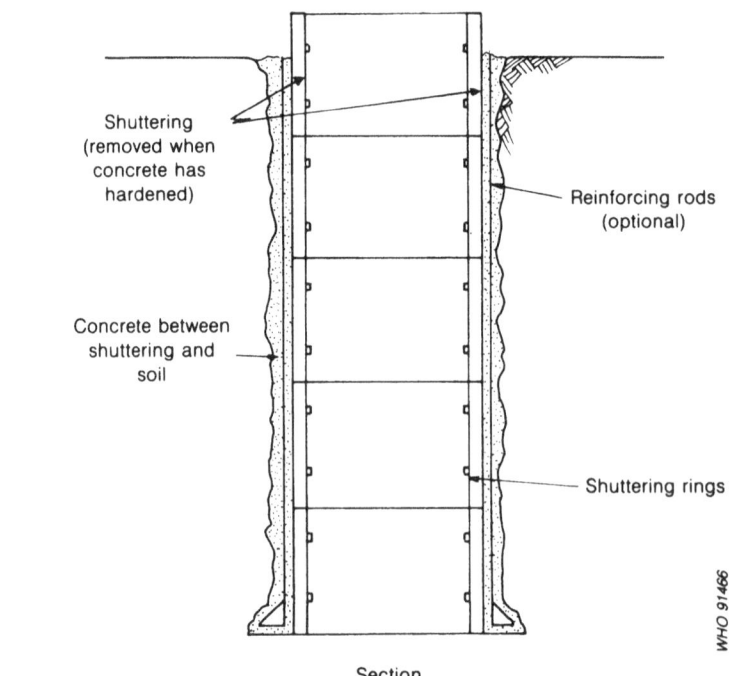

Section

the lining. Except for the top 300–500 mm, the joints are left open as described above to ensure infiltration of liquid to the soil.

*In situ concrete lining*

In this method the hole is lined with concrete cast in the hole (Fig. 7.6). After excavation, shuttering is positioned to a convenient height

**Fig. 7.6. Pit with concrete lining *in situ***

Section

allowing for compaction, and the space between is filled with concrete. Normally the concrete does not require steel reinforcement for structural strength. However, a small amount of steel may reduce shrinkage cracking. The lining can be made porous by leaving small holes in the concrete (short lengths of 25–50 mm of pipe fitted between the shuttering and the soil will be satisfactory). Alternatively "no fines" concrete can be used.

*Ferrocement lining*

When mortar is plastered over layers of fine wire mesh (such as chicken wire) the resulting material is called ferrocement. It is strong, light, requires no shuttering and is easy to construct. It is now widely used for such structures as water tanks and latrine slabs and can be adapted for use as a pit lining.

In some countries the term ferrocement refers to any cement-based material reinforced with steel. Specifically it now describes a material consisting of several layers of small-diameter steel mesh (usually hexagonal chicken wire, with wire of 0.7–1.3 mm in diameter and openings of 12 mm). The layers are tied together with fine wire at 150-mm intervals and then plastered with a rich cement mortar (one volume of cement to two volumes of sand) to give a finished thickness of about 25 mm.

After excavating the hole, as much loose material as possible is removed from the pit walls. Cement mortar is applied directly to the walls of the pit to give a layer approximately 12 mm thick. This layer is then covered with two or three thicknesses of steel mesh, held in place with long staples driven through the mortar into the soil. A second coat of mortar is then applied and pushed firmly into the holes in the wire mesh. On completion, the mortar covering the mesh should be at least 10 mm thick. Where a porous lining is required, holes can be punched through the mortar while it is still weak.

Ferrocement rings may also be precast on the surface and used in the same way as concrete rings.

## Excavation in loose ground

Where the ground is very loose and liable to collapse if left unsupported, or where the excavation enters the water table, the most common method of construction is to prefabricate the lining on the surface, place it in a starter excavation, dig out the soil below and allow the lining to sink as the hole is dug. This method is called "caissoning" (Fig. 7.7).

A hole is excavated as deep as possible (experience of the local ground conditions will determine the depth). A precast concrete ring fitted with a cutting edge is then placed in the hole. Additional rings are placed on top until ground level is reached. Excavation now begins inside the rings. As the ground is dug away from under the cutting

**Fig. 7.7. "Caissoning" a pit**

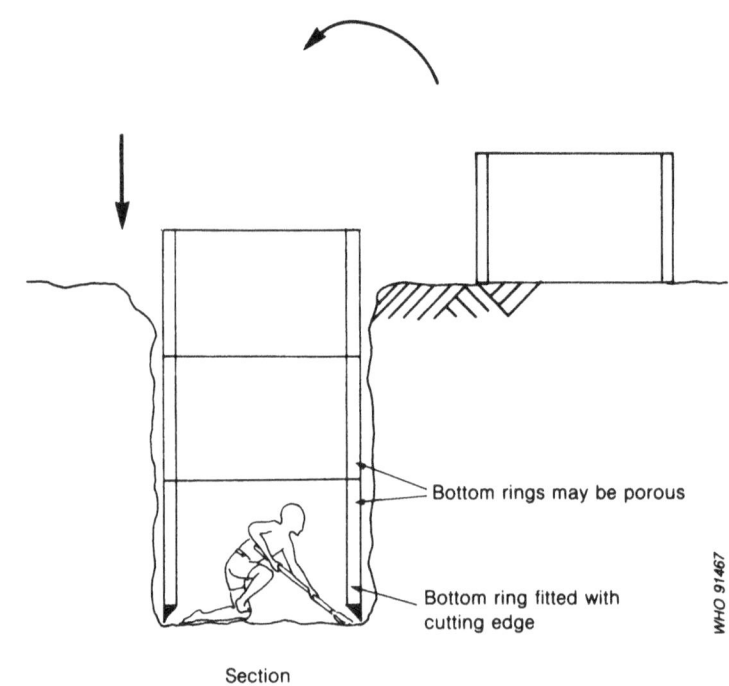

Bottom rings may be porous

Bottom ring fitted with
cutting edge

WHO 91467

Section

edge, the rings start to sink under their own weight. Additional rings are then placed on top until the required depth is reached.

This method may also be used for linings of bricks or blocks. However, the lining must be constructed sufficiently far above the ground to ensure that the mortar has fully set before the lining enters the ground. The honeycomb method of construction cannot normally be expected to have sufficient strength to be sunk as a caisson.

Where caissoning is employed because of a high groundwater table, excavation should take place towards the end of the dry season when the water table is at its lowest. As the lower ring enters the water it is possible to continue excavation for up to one metre by scooping material in a bucket or with a specially shaped shovel.

### Backfilling

Any space around the outside of the lining should be backfilled with compacted earth taken from the pit or, where available, with sand and gravel. If the ground is particularly weak, the top of the pit may be backfilled with weak concrete or a soil-cement mixture to give additional strength. Strengthening may be important if the top of the pit has become overly enlarged during excavation.

## Latrine floors

Floors of latrines, whether laid on the ground or supported over a pit, should be smooth and impervious so that they may be cleaned easily and have a satisfactory appearance to users. The upper surface should be at least 150 mm above the surrounding ground level (Fig. 7.8) to prevent rain and surface water entering the latrine.

The floor surface should slope gently to facilitate cleaning and to prevent surplus wash water from collecting in puddles. The slope is normally from the outer edge of the floor towards the squat hole or pan at the centre, so that the water used for cleaning flows into the pit and does not foul the area surrounding the slab. A fall of about 20 mm between the edge and the centre of a slab up to 1.5 m across is sufficient to prevent pools of liquid forming (Fig. 7.8). Where seats are used, the floor should slope away from the seat support so that any wash water flows towards the latrine entrance.

If a precast slab is smaller than the inside floor area of the superstructure, an impervious surface is normally provided to seal the area between the slab and the inside wall of the building. Any area around the slab which is left as bare earth could be fouled, thus becoming a possible site for hookworm infestation. However, in order to minimize costs, the space around the squatting area inside the superstructure should be limited. This reduces building costs for the superstructure as well as flooring materials. But the squat hole or pan should not be so close to the superstructure that users are forced to lean against the wall when they are trying to defecate. A minimum floor space of 80 cm in width and 1 m from front to back is normally acceptable (Mara, 1985b).

## Slabs

### Requirements

A latrine slab serves two main purposes, as a support and as a seal. It has to support the weight of the person using the latrine and, possibly, the

**Fig. 7.8. Requirements of slabs**

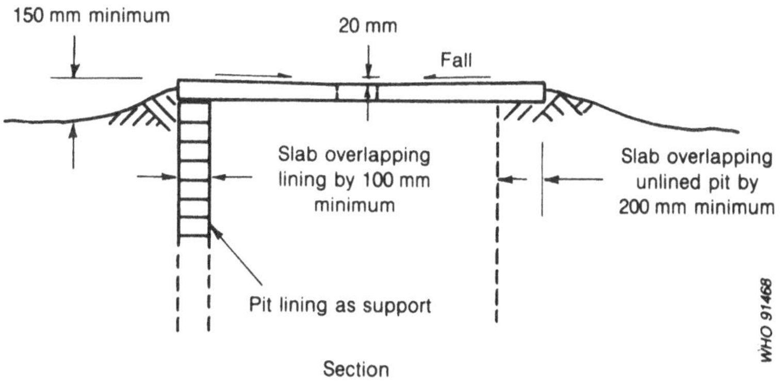

150 mm minimum

20 mm

Fall

Slab overlapping lining by 100 mm minimum

Slab overlapping unlined pit by 200 mm minimum

Pit lining as support

Section

WHO 91468

weight of the superstructure. It also seals the pit, with the exception of the squat hole and, where required, the vent-pipe hole. This facilitates control of flies and smells and reduces the likelihood of rodents and surface water entering the pit. Where the slab has been made in sections (for ease of placing and emptying) or has a removable cover, the joints should be sealed with a weak mortar such as a lime or mud mortar.

To support the weight of a person over a latrine pit the suspended slab has to act structurally in the manner of a bridge. Where seats are provided, the extra weight has to be allowed for when designing the slab. Depending on the design of the slab, the materials may have to be able to resist forces in tension as well as in compression (Fig. 7.9). The materials needed to carry the tensile forces are often more expensive than those commonly used in low-cost buildings. The slab is often the most expensive individual component that has to be paid for by the user. It is therefore important to ensure that it is carefully designed to serve its purpose with a minimum of costly material.

The slab normally rests on a foundation or on the top of the pit lining (see Fig. 7.8). This ensures that the weight of the slab and the weight of the person using it are spread evenly on the soil. Particular care must be taken where the slab also has to carry part of the weight of the superstructure. If the ground is weak, the foundation prevents subsidence or collapse of the ground underneath the load. Any gaps between the slab and the pit lining should be sealed with earth or a weak mortar to prevent ingress of water. This seal also prevents small animals and insects getting into and out of the pit.

Where a pit is excavated to a larger diameter than planned, precast slabs are occasionally supported on timber poles. This practice is not advisable as the heavy load on the poles is likely to lead to early failure.

**Fig. 7.9. Tension and compression forces in a slab**

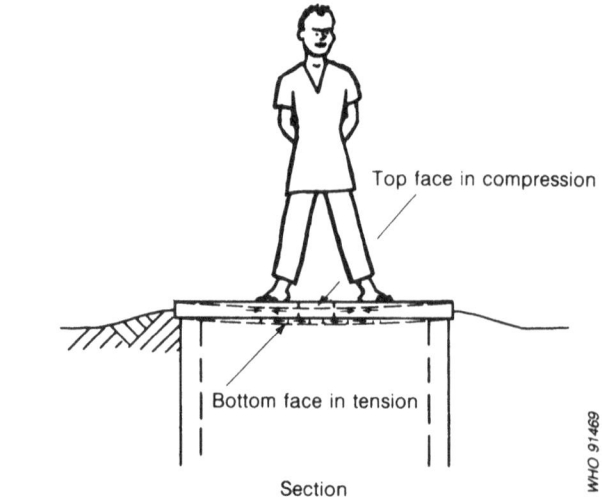

Top face in compression

Bottom face in tension

Section

WHO 91469

**Fig. 7.10. Small slabs for upgrading timber and earth structures**

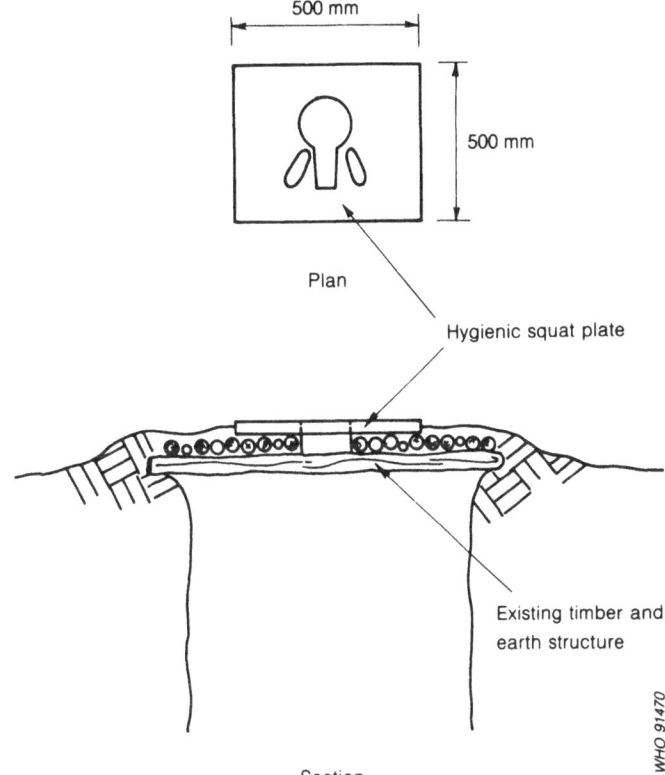

However, small slabs (approximately 500 mm square), designed to provide a hygienic squat hole for existing latrines at minimum cost, will not overload a timber support (Fig. 7.10).

The latrine slab should feel secure and should not deflect noticeably under the weight of a person using the latrine. It needs to be as clean and attractive as possible so that people feel comfortable using the latrine. There is then much less chance of the latrine being misused or fouled.

Offset pits used with pour-flush latrines require a cover slab to prevent entry of flies and rodents and to ensure safety, particularly of children. With the omission of a squat hole, the structural requirements are the same as for a latrine slab.

## Shapes of direct pit slabs

The shape and size of the pit are the first factors to be considered when designing a supported slab. Latrine pits can be round, square or rectangular and it is usual to find that a particular shape becomes the accepted design for a particular area.

Borehole latrines have a small span and therefore require very simple slabs. The shape will depend on the users' needs for a clean hygienic area with correctly spaced footrests, rather than being controlled by the size of the hole to be covered. Larger, hand-dug pits 1–1.5 m in width require a shape designed to span and seal the pit. An exception to this is where the span of the slab is reduced by corbelling the top of the lining (Fig. 7.11). This decreases the amount of material required in the slab and thus reduces the cost.

**Fig. 7.11. Minimizing the span of the slab**

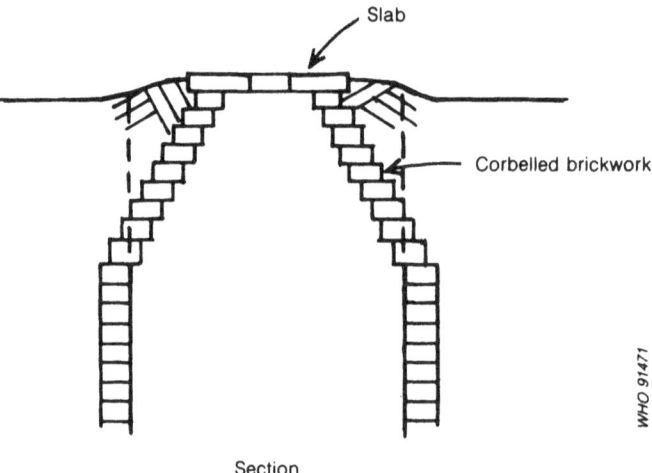

Section

Slabs may be precast or constructed *in situ*, which means that the slabs are built over the pit, exactly where they are to be used. In a large agency-assisted programme, slabs are often manufactured at a convenient construction site away from the latrines and then brought to the site and laid across the pits. Where slabs are to be moved, weight and shape are both significant factors.

The shape of the slab is also determined by the type of latrine. Water-seal latrines, aqua-privies, ventilated pits and pits sealed with hole covers all have different requirements. For example, the need for an extra hole close to the edge of the slab for a vent pipe makes the unreinforced dome slab unsuitable for ventilated latrines.

The slab normally overlaps the supporting pit lining or foundation by at least 100 mm on all sides to ensure that the load is adequately transferred. This overlap may have to be extended to 200 mm where the pit is unlined and the slab is resting directly on the soil (see Fig. 7.8).

## Cement-based slabs and components

In most countries, concrete or cement-based slabs provide the most durable and economic method of covering latrine pits. There are many different ways of using cement. Its ability to bind with other materials and provide a clean watertight surface make it the obvious choice for the majority of programmes.

Concrete is a mixture of cement, sand, gravel and water. When set, it forms a hard dense material which is extremely strong in compression but weak in tension. Cast as a simple flat slab across a pit, its own weight and the weight of any person on it forces the concrete to deflect downwards in the centre. As the load increases, small tension cracks form on the underside of the beam. With heavy loads, these cracks may extend upwards through the concrete until the slab breaks. To prevent this happening, steel bars or other reinforcement may be placed in the concrete on the lower side of the slab to carry the tension load and prevent the cracks spreading.

### Unreinforced concrete

Small slabs, such as those required for borehole latrines or to provide a hygienic platform for the squatting area of timber-supported slabs (see Fig. 7.10), do not need any reinforcement. Where an unreinforced span of greater than 0.5 m is required, the slab should be cast in the form of a "flat" arch. The weight of the load is then directed through the arch to the supporting area on the ground. The underside of the concrete remains in compression and no reinforcement is required. Using this principle, a shallow circular dome or arch can be constructed to cover a latrine pit. The dome is strong enough to support itself and the people using it without any expensive steel reinforcement. A slab using this principle has been developed by a team in Mozambique (Fig. 7.12) and

**Fig. 7.12. Dimensions of domed slab without reinforcement**

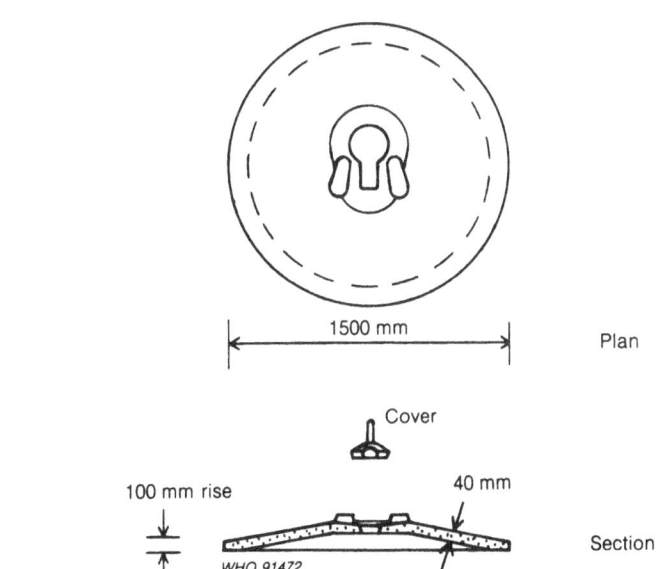

has proved to be economical and popular. The slabs are about 40 mm thick and rise 100 mm in the centre to give the arch effect (International Development Research Centre, 1983).

Although such domed slabs fall away from the centre, a small inward slope about 100 mm wide immediately around the squat hole is incorporated to direct any waste into the pit. These slabs have been used most effectively in areas with sandy soil which quickly absorbs any surplus wash water.

The concrete slab is given the shape of a dome by mounding up earth to the required profile of the underside of the slab. The earth is compacted and smoothed. It may then be covered with plastic sheeting or old cement bags, or coated in old engine oil to break any bond between the earth and the fresh concrete. A circular iron strip made from an oil drum is used as the edge former or mould. The concrete around the centre hole is made slightly thinner so that a slope towards the hole can be made. Each slab has to be allowed to harden undisturbed for several days after casting.

To save space in the casting yard, up to five slabs may be cast on top of each other, using a lower, previously cast slab as a former for the next slab. Particular attention has to be given to the concrete mix of a thin unreinforced slab. A maximum aggregate size of 10 mm and slightly more cement than usual is required. The recommended mix is one part by volume of cement to two parts of sand and one and a half parts of 6–10 mm aggregate.

An unreinforced slab may also be produced in a rectangular mould with a flat upper surface and a dome on the underside (Fig. 7.13). As an

**Fig. 7.13. Semi-domed slab**

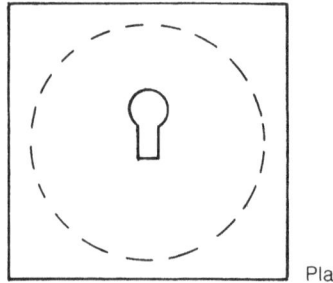

Plan

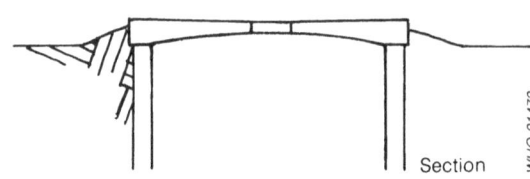

Section

WHO 91473

**Fig. 7.14. Arched brickwork lining and support**

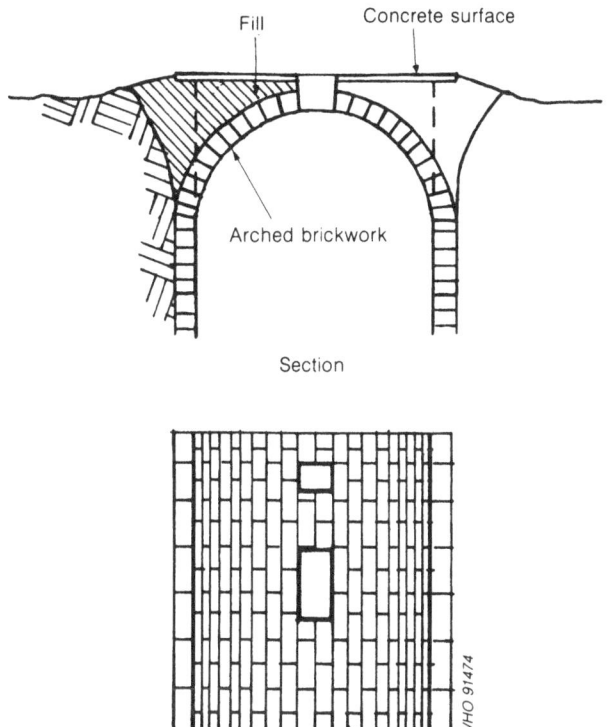

unreinforced dome slab cannot accept a second hole close to one edge for a vent pipe, flies, smells and cockroaches are prevented from leaving the pit by providing a tight-fitting cover over the squat hole. This is cast directly in the squat hole so that it fits exactly. A layer of cement bag paper may be used to prevent the fresh concrete sticking to the old.

Bricks can be used to form an unreinforced arch across a rectangular pit (Fig. 7.14) using a rough framework of bamboo, reeds or forest poles which is left in the pit. The space above the arch is levelled with river sand and topped with a 20-mm cement–sand screed sloping towards the centre. This technique requires very little cement and no steel. However, these structures have to be built by skilled masons and there is no opportunity for precasting. Emptying of the pit can only be carried out through the squat hole.

### Reinforced concrete

Because of the weakness of concrete in tension it is often reinforced with other materials. Most commonly it is strengthened by the inclusion of steel bars. Details of the reinforcing steel required for common sizes of slab are shown in Table 7.1. Mild steel bars, 6 mm in diameter

**Table 7.1. Spacing of steel reinforcement bars for concrete slabs**[a]

| Slab thickness (mm) | Steel bar diameter (mm) | Spacing of steel bars (mm) for minimum slab span of: | | | | |
|---|---|---|---|---|---|---|
| | | 1 m | 1.25 m | 1.5 m | 1.75 m | 2 m |
| 65 | 6 | 150 | 150 | 125 | 75 | 50 |
| | 8 | 250 | 250 | 200 | 150 | 125 |
| 80 | 6 | 150 | 150 | 150 | 125 | 75 |
| | 8 | 250 | 250 | 250 | 200 | 150 |

[a] The steel bars should be fixed on the lower side of the slab, with 12-mm cover or thickness of concrete beneath each bar. Steel to be laid at above spacings in both directions. Size and spacing of steel calculated for grade 20 concrete and mild steel reinforcement, with characteristic yield stress of 210 N/mm², or high-yield mesh, yield stress 485 N/mm².

spaced at intervals of 150 mm, or 8 mm in diameter spaced at intervals of 250 mm in each direction, are normally sufficient for 80-mm thick slabs of up to 1.5 m in span. This span distance is measured at the point of minimum span, that is, the shortest distance between two points which fully support the slab. Where used correctly, reinforcement in a concrete slab will support at least six adults on a 1.5-m span slab. For the small spans illustrated, extra steel is not required for trimming around the pit opening.

The reinforcing steel is laid in both directions, that is, with one layer of bars perpendicular to the second layer (Fig. 7.15). Where the slab is rectangular, the bars parallel to the direction of the minimum

**Fig. 7.15. Reinforced concrete rectangular slab (for details of reinforcement see Table 7.1)**

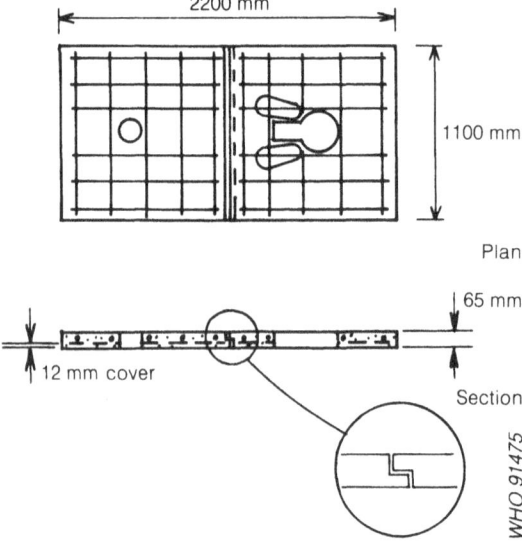

100

span should be beneath the bars in the direction of the longer span. For the bars specified, a characteristic yield strength for the steel of 210 N/mm² is assumed. Care is required to ensure that the steel is of the required quality.

When individual bars are used, some may be omitted by mistake. One way of avoiding this is to use steel mesh, which consists of smaller-diameter bars welded together. This can be cut to the required shape but there is likely to be wastage of the off-cuts that have to be discarded. A mesh with 7-mm bars at 200-mm centres, with a cross-sectional steel area of 193 mm²/m (yield stress 485 N/mm²) is normally sufficient.

Care must be taken when reinforcing concrete with steel to ensure that the steel is completely surrounded by the concrete. There should be at least 12 mm of concrete under the steel bars and at the ends of all bars. This protects the steel from the corrosive effect of gases and moisture in the pit. When concrete is placed in a mould or former it has to be compacted by manual or mechanical vibration to remove any air bubbles and to ensure the durability of the completed slab. Simple wooden or steel moulds can be reused many times to give the required shape to the wet concrete if they are coated with a suitable release agent. There are many proprietary agents, but used engine oil painted on to the mould effectively prevents the concrete from sticking. Alternatively, plastic sheeting or empty cement bags may be used to prevent bonding. These materials may also be used between the ground and the underside of the slab. The squat hole is formed using a shaped wooden mould with a bevelled edge. A vent pipe opening may be created with an offcut of plastic pipe which is removed a few hours after casting so that it can be reused many times.

An alternative way of using steel for reinforcement is to precast a ferrocement slab. The method of construction is described under construction of linings, p. 89. A flat ferrocement slab is strong enough to carry the imposed load but is too flexible for the users' comfort. In order to ensure adequate stiffness, the ferrocement may be shaped as a dome or may be cast with ribs on the soffit (Fig. 7.16). Four layers of mesh are normally required for a slab with a 1-m span. It is necessary to ensure that the cement mortar has been adequately pressed through all the layers of wire mesh and compacted to a dense material if it is to have adequate strength.

Steel reinforcement is used in various ways in different countries reflecting differences in price and availability. Because of the relatively high cost of steel, many techniques have been investigated in the search for cheaper alternatives. One approach is to reinforce concrete with small unconnected fibres with a low modulus of elasticity. These are either natural fibres, such as sisal, jute, coir, Manila hemp or kenaf, or man-made fibres such as fibrillated polypropylene. The fibres are chopped and added to the cement mix. Use of these low-modulus fibres does not reinforce the concrete in the conventional sense of carrying the tensile load, but is particularly beneficial in ensuring adequate curing of the concrete without the formation of minute shrinkage cracks (Parry,

**Fig. 7.16. Ferrocement slab**

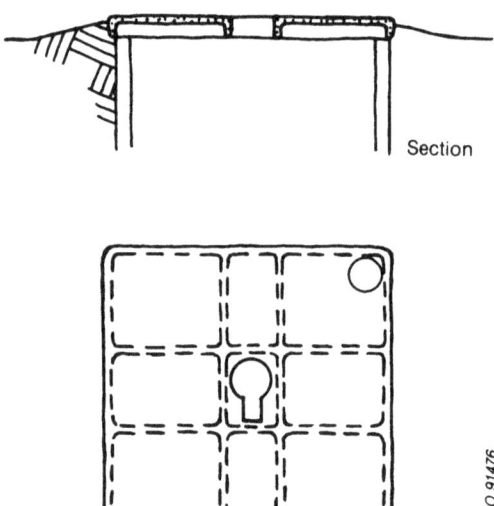

1985). The resultant "unreinforced" concrete attains a much higher tensile strength than would otherwise be possible. Slabs made from fibre-reinforced cement should normally be given the shape of an arch or dome to minimize tensile forces in the soffit.

Slabs have also been reinforced with barbed wire, fencing wire, scrap steel from cars and broken machinery, redundant universal beams and almost anything that is available. Although a saving is made on reinforcement, these methods usually lead to a much greater use of concrete in order to cover the larger sections of steel and therefore are rarely economical.

Bamboo has a high strength-to-weight ratio and in certain parts of the world is widely available. Because of the low cost, bamboo strips have been used as an alternative to steel bars but it is important to ensure that the bamboo strips in a slab are completely covered by the concrete so that water and vapours cannot rot the bamboo. The strips should initially be treated with preservative. One recommended method (UNCHS, undated) is for the bamboo to be dipped in white lead and 10% varnish to inhibit water absorption from the freshly placed concrete. Even where treated, there is some doubt as to the long-term durability of bamboo as reinforcement.

Where cement is relatively expensive, a technique known as re-inforced brickwork can be utilized, in which part of the concrete is replaced by whole or half bricks, leaving steel reinforced concrete ribs to support the bricks (Fig. 7.17). The whole slab requires a cement skimming over the surface to make it impervious to fouling by the users.

**Fig. 7.17. Reinforced brickwork slab**

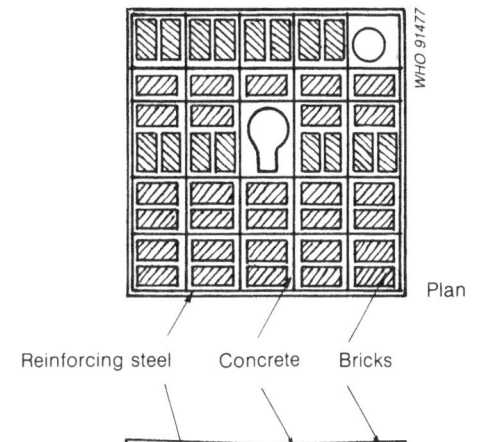

Reinforcing steel    Concrete    Bricks

Plan

Section

## Concrete mixes

Different concrete design mixes (that is, combinations of cement, sand, aggregate and water) are suitable for use in various circumstances. The concrete mix that is most often used is 1:2:4 (one unit by volume of cement with two units by volume of sand and four units by volume of aggregate). The sand should be clean and hard and may be sized by sieving through ordinary mosquito netting. Coarse aggregate comprises graded stones 6–18 mm in size and should be free of fine dust. This mix results in a finished volume of concrete which is approximately 70% of the total volume of the individual dry materials.

The cement, sand and coarse aggregate have to be mixed with a specific amount of water to give the optimum strength for the amount of cement used. For concrete mixed and placed by hand, there should normally be a water:cement ratio of 0.55 by weight, i.e., the weight of water is approximately half the weight of cement. Cement weighs 1400 kg/m³ and water 1000 kg/m³; a 50-kg bag of cement thus has a volume of 0.035 m³. A 1:2:4 concrete mix using one 50-kg bag of cement therefore requires 0.070 m³ of clean sand, 0.140 m³ of aggregate and 0.027 m³ of water, which results in 0.17 m³ of finished concrete.

The volume of water is applicable where the aggregate and sand are "saturated, surface dry". In hot dry climates, the small pores in the aggregate, as well as the surface, are likely to be "oven dry" rather than saturated. To use the specified amount of water would then lead to an extremely stiff, unworkable concrete. The aggregate should therefore be thoroughly wetted with water before mixing begins. The correct water:cement ratio results in a relatively stiff but workable material which produces a skim of water on the surface of the concrete as it is worked flat with a trowel. When the mix has too much water, the

**Fig. 7.18. Checking the water content of concrete with a slump cone**

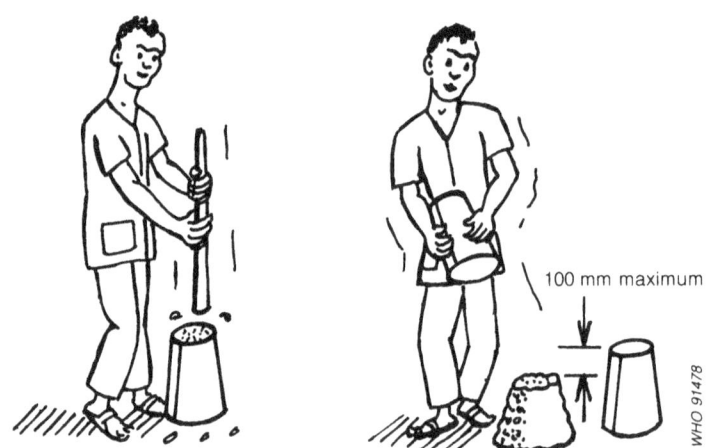

strength is reduced considerably. An increase of only 50% in the water content decreases the finished concrete strength by half, which is the equivalent of wasting half the cement in the bag.

To check that the calculated amount of water is correct, a trial mix may be prepared and a slump test carried out. In this test, the concrete mix is compacted into a slump cone (Fig. 7.18), which is similar to an upturned bucket 300 mm high with the base removed. When the cone is removed, the concrete will slump, i.e., reduce in height; the maximum slump, for concrete that is to be reinforced, should be about 100 mm, and less for unreinforced concrete.

### Caring for concrete

After it has been cast, concrete must be cured. It should be covered with either wet sand, straw, cement bags, jute sacks, plastic or palm leaves to keep the concrete moist and as cool as possible. The chemical reaction which causes the cement particles to bind is dependent upon the amount of water present. If the moisture has been sucked out from the surface of the concrete by the heat of the sun, the chemical reaction cannot take place and the surface of the slab will not be durable. In hot dry climates the concrete and its covering need to be watered twice a day for seven days after casting. If the concrete is not cured, it will have only 60% of its ultimate design strength; if cured for three days, it will attain only 80%, but if kept damp for seven days will reach almost 100% (Reynolds & Steedman, 1974).

A good guide for field workers is: "Make the concrete mixture as dry as you can; and then keep the cast concrete as wet as you can."

The most effective way of checking the strength of a slab is to test load it seven days after casting. As, normally, only one person at a time will use the latrine, to test load the slab with five or six people gives an adequate and convincing factor of safety. The slab should be supported at its edges by four or five bricks placed on flat ground, and the people should stand on the slab, avoiding areas directly over the bricks. Testing the strength of precast slabs by throwing them off the back of the delivery truck at the site, on the understanding that those that do not break are adequate, is not recommended.

The final concrete surface should be clean, dense and free of blemishes. The surface will absorb urine unless it is sealed effectively with, for example, proprietary sealant, alkali-resistant gloss paint, bitumastic paint, or two coats of a 25% solution of silicate of soda (Khanna, 1985).

A screed (a thin layer of cement mortar) is sometimes applied to a flat slab after casting to create the desired slope towards the squat hole. However, unless the screed is applied before the concrete has completely set there is a danger of its flaking off in use. Wherever possible the required slope should be cast in the original concrete, a dense surface being obtained by trowelling with a steel float as the concrete begins to set. Alternatively the slab may be cast upside down on plastic sheeting to ensure a good finish.

Footrests are normally cast separately, after the concrete of the slab has hardened. The area where the rests will be cast is roughened when the slab surface is being given its final trowelling. Formers for the footrests can be made out of any available material such as tin or wood, but the individual formers should be connected together and to fixed points on the edge of the slab to ensure that the rests are always cast in the same position (Fig. 7.19).

**Fig. 7.19. Formwork for the casting of footrests**

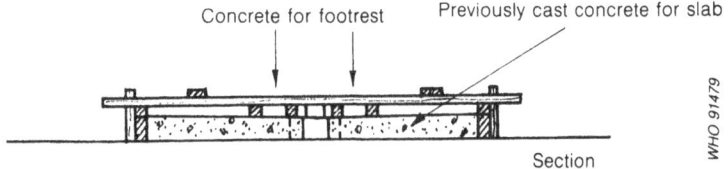

Footrest former

Concrete slab

Slab former

Plan

Fixing of footrest formers to slab former to ensure uniformity

Concrete for footrest

Previously cast concrete for slab

Section

WHO 91479

### *Weights of concrete slabs*

If cement-based slabs are to be moved, weight is an important consideration. For example, a 65-mm-thick circular concrete slab, 1.5 m in diameter, weighs approximately 275 kg, while an 80-mm thick slab weighs 340 kg. A rectangular slab, 65 mm thick, designed to cover a pit of size 2.2 m × 1.1 m would weigh 360 kg, unless made in sections (Fig. 7.20). Circular slabs are not normally made in sections. When whole, a round slab can be moved by two or three people, rolling it on its edge (Fig. 7.21). This is particularly useful in the management of the construction yard and can sometimes even be used to transfer the slab to the household site without a vehicle.

**Fig. 7.20. Rectangular slab in two sections**

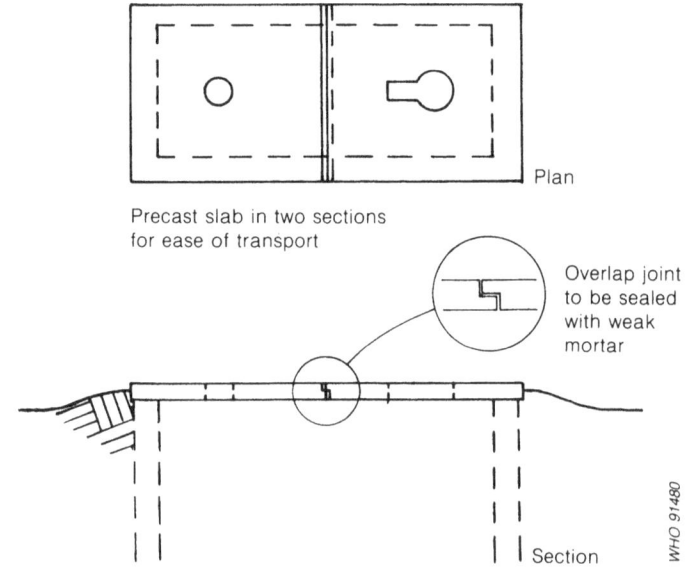

**Fig. 7.21. Circular slab for ease of transport**

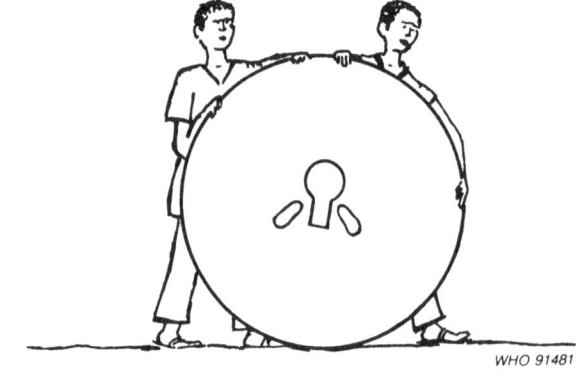

### Concrete for other components

Concrete for floors of latrines that are not directly above the pits is cast *in situ*. A slightly weaker concrete mix of 1:3:6 may be used but the curing requirements remain as described above. The outlet pipe and pan should be carefully laid to the desired level before the concrete is cast.

Cover slabs for offset pits and floors and cover slabs of septic tanks are normally also made of concrete. Walls of septic tanks are usually constructed from concrete blocks or cement-plastered fired bricks. The requirements for good quality concrete are identical to those for components discussed previously.

## Other materials for slabs

### Wood

The simplest slabs in rural areas are made from rough poles and tree branches laid closely together over the pit. A timber slab is always liable to deterioration because of fungal decay owing to the moist gases rising from the pit and also because of the threat from termites and boring insects in tropical climates. Durable timbers such as the heartwood of some tropical hardwoods are normally too expensive for use in latrines but, where available, may be expected to last satisfactorily for several years.

A thick layer of earth or mud is often spread over the poles or branches to bind them together and create a smooth surface (Fig. 7.22). In many places, people are skilled at making mud floors which are almost as hard as cement and quite smooth. They need not be rough or unsanitary. There are various methods of improving the mud with local materials, such as mixing the soil with a liquor obtained by soaking animal dung overnight. In some areas the mud is mixed with charcoal or other small aggregate, or with cow dung and then smeared with ashes. Alternatively, the mud from ant-hills has been found to make a hard, practically waterproof surface (Denyer, 1978). If the surface is not kept in good condition, however, there is a danger of hookworm larvae penetrating the feet of users.

The life of a rough timber slab can be extended by using a mixture of soil and cement to plaster and protect the wood. Alternatively, a thin cement mortar screed can be laid over the surface of the earth to protect against hookworm and to improve hygiene. However, it is usually more cost-effective to use the cement to provide a permanent concrete slab which can be transferred to a new pit when the first is filled. Where more than half a bag of cement is needed to stabilize the earth, a concrete slab is likely to be a cheaper alternative.

In an area where timber is abundant, hewn or sawn logs supporting a platform of wooden planks make a floor that is preferable to the mud and pole version (Fig. 7.23). The surface can be kept clean, and signs of

**Fig. 7.22. Timber and earth slab**

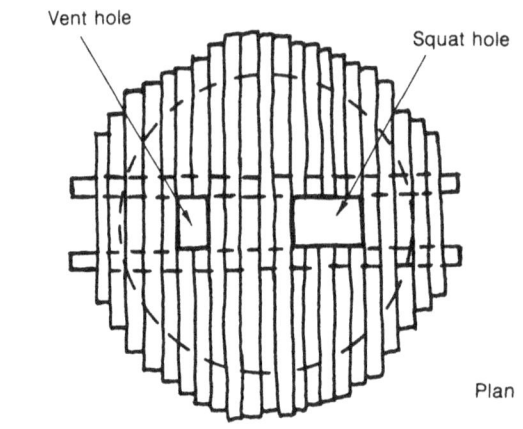

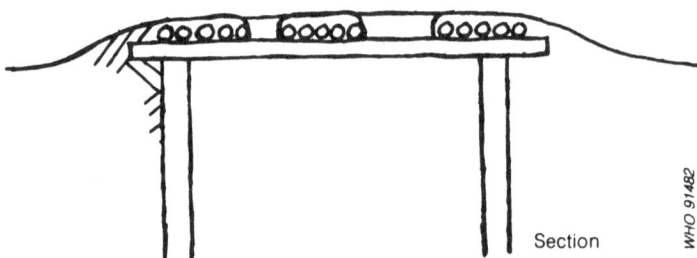

imminent collapse are normally apparent to the adult user. The durability of timbers may be improved by some form of treatment. The effectiveness of these treatments depends upon the amount of preservative that the timber can be made to absorb, which is a function of the permeability of the timber and the process used. Suitable preservatives include ordinary tar, tar-oils such as creosote, water-based preservatives such as copper/chrome/arsenic, and specialized organic solvents (Tack, 1979). Each type of preservative has its own characteristics and particular uses. Where treated timber is not available and the cost of using preservatives on a small scale is high, other more durable alternatives may be cheaper in the long run.

Simple timber slabs are often considered to be unsuitable for sanitation projects, since people are less likely to use the latrine if they are afraid that the slab may collapse under them. However, the danger of collapse is usually less than the dangers associated with not having any appropriate system of sanitation. If no other materials are available at reasonable cost, a rough pole slab that has to be renewed every few years is to be preferred to no latrine at all.

**Fig. 7.23. Sawn timber slab**

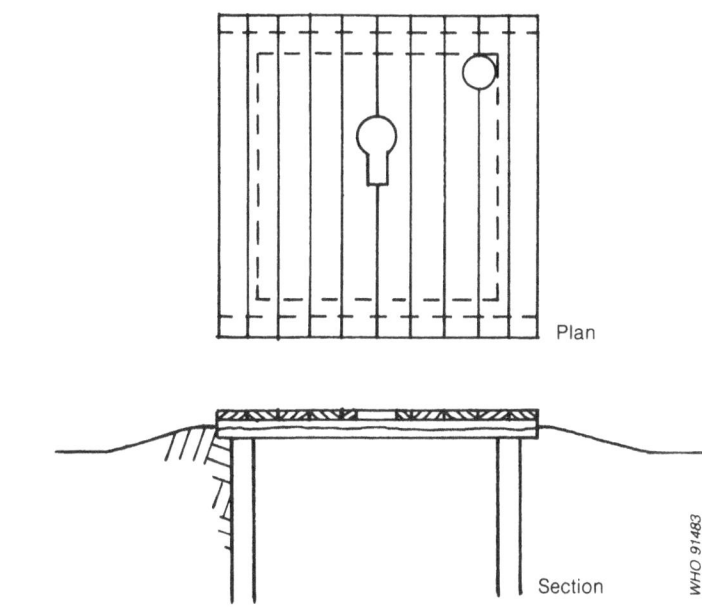

Plan

Section

WHO 91483

### Scrap iron and steel

In urban areas where sanitation is most urgently required, supplies of even the cheapest materials, such as rough poles, are usually limited and relatively expensive. The simplest alternative used by householders on an informal basis is to lay parts of discarded vehicles or any other scrap materials across the pit opening to provide support, with flattened containers, oil drums or galvanized iron roofing sheet to make a surface. Such materials do not seal the pit but they enable the user to excrete into a relatively safe hole rather than at the side of the street. However, where there are significant dangers, especially for children, these methods cannot be recommended.

### Miscellaneous materials

Slabs have been made in a variety of other materials. Glass-reinforced plastics, polyvinyl chloride (PVC), ceramics and glass fibre have all been used to meet particular needs and situations. Plastic floors tend to flex under the weight of the user unless they are deeply ribbed. Some of these materials can also be used to give a special surface finish to concrete slabs.

## Footrests and squat holes

Footrests are required to lift the users' feet off the slab in case it is already fouled and also to position the users so that they are less likely to dirty the slab or the edge of the squat hole. The positions and sizes of footrests must be determined to suit the needs of the people in each area. Fig. 7.24 indicates a typical layout. Different people in different societies with different-sized bodies and varying flexibility of tendons may excrete between their feet or behind their ankles. Their feet may be parallel or angled. It is therefore advisable to check with young and old, and with male and female in a community before assuming a particular layout. McClelland & Ward (1976) reported that in one sample of 140 people, the distance from heel to anus in a squatting adult varied from 0 to 0.25 m with a mean of 0.13 m for men and 0.10 m for women.

Excreta enter a pit either by falling through a squat hole or by passing through a water seal. Details of seals are given later. Squat holes have to be large enough to limit fouling of the edges but not so large that children are frightened of using the latrine. The hole can either be rectangular, elliptical, pear-shaped or circular with a straight extension as in a keyhole (Fig. 7.25). The maximum width should be 180 mm and the length at least 350 mm. In a concrete slab, the edge of the former used to make the hole should be angled to ease its withdrawal after casting.

**Fig. 7.24. Possible footrest positions**

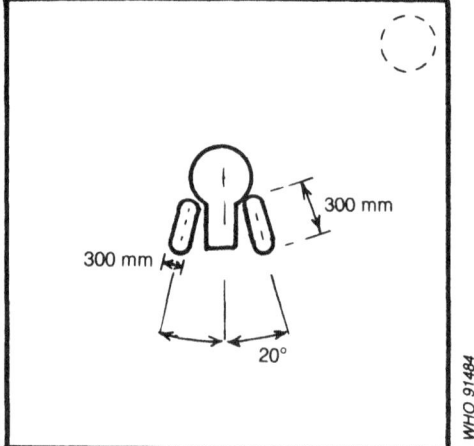

## Seats for latrines

In many parts of the world, people prefer to sit to defecate. To make a latrine seat, a support or pedestal is built or mounted on top of the slab. The seat level should be at a position that is comfortable for the majority of the users (Fig. 7.26); this is normally about 350 mm above the top of the slab.

The seat support can be made on site from brick, concrete, mud block or timber and should be designed to minimize the load on the

**Fig. 7.25. Squat hole shapes and former**

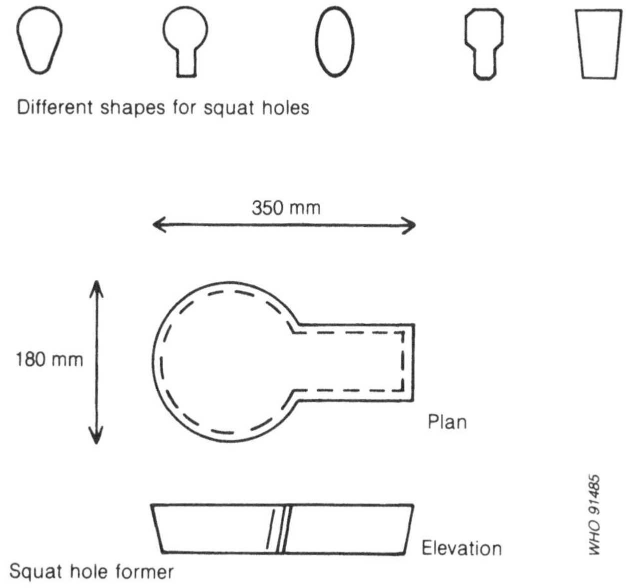

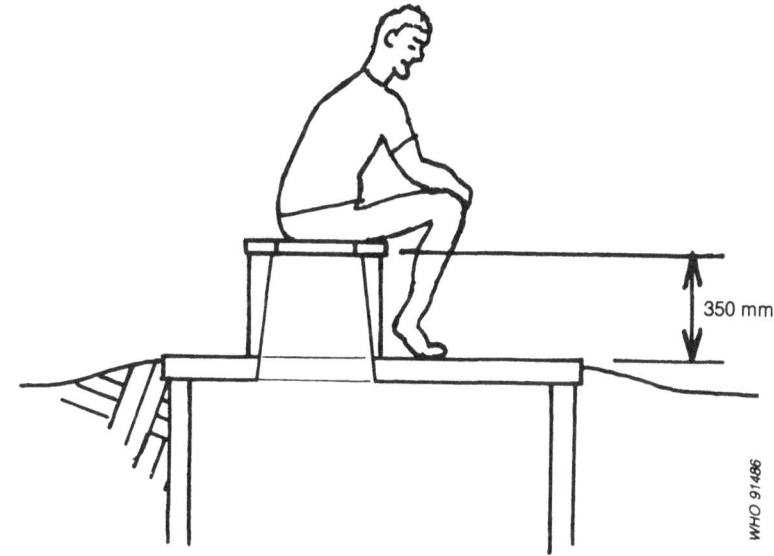

Different shapes for squat holes

350 mm

180 mm

Plan

Squat hole former          Elevation

WHO 91485

**Fig. 7.26. Latrine seat**

350 mm

WHO 91486

slab. A heavy type of construction adds weight to the slab which then requires more expensive reinforcement to carry the load. Commercially available or project-manufactured pedestals made of ceramic, glass-reinforced plastic (GRP), PVC or ferrocement can also be used where people can afford them.

111

**Fig. 7.27. Pedestal seat liner**

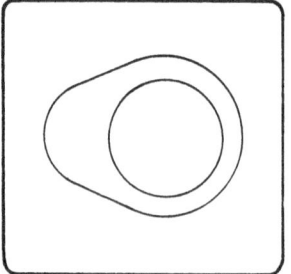

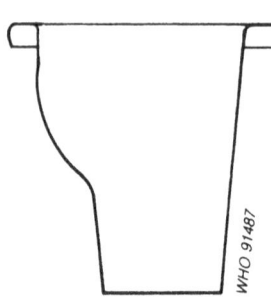

The inside of the pedestal should be designed to prevent constant fouling by excreta, which leads to increased odour and fly breeding. One approach is to use a large-diameter opening of 250 mm or more, but this might discourage use by children who are frightened by the large opening. An alternative is to have a 180-mm diameter hole through the pedestal which is lined with a smooth material such as cement mortar or an insert of glass fibre (Fig. 7.27) or ceramic. A third alternative is a tapered hole, increasing from an opening size of about 180 mm at seat level to 300 mm at the slab. If possible the pedestal should overhang slightly so that the seat can be used with the feet tucked under to mimic the squatting position.

Shapes of locally made pedestals vary from a rectangular box, where the user sits on one side but can also sit across a corner with one foot on either side, to a circular or oval design. It is important to obtain a good seal between the pedestal and the slab.

A seat cover may be fitted to seal off an unventilated pit. Where a vent pipe is fitted, an adequate flow of air to the pit can be obtained by raising the seat cover slightly above the seat, as is the case with conventional flush pedestals.

A special fitment with a small opening can be made to encourage children to use the latrine. Alternatively the pedestal top can be enlarged to accommodate a second seat with a smaller opening, possibly at a lower level, for the use of children.

## Water seals and pans

A pour-flush latrine utilizes a water seal to prevent odour and insects entering the latrine from the pit. This water seal may be part of the pan unit (Fig. 7.28) or may be connected immediately below the pan (Fig. 7. 29). For on-site sanitation, flushing is normally carried out by the wash-down method where the force of the flush water thrown into the pan is enough to drive the excreta through the water seal.

The pan may be of the squatting type or of the pedestal variety where the user can sit. The amount of water needed for flushing

**Fig. 7.28. Combined pan and water seal for direct pour-flush latrine**

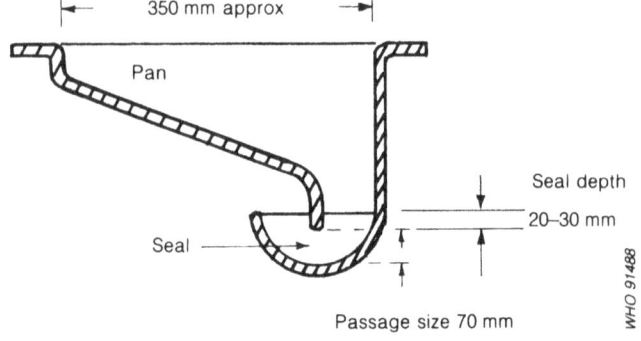

**Fig. 7.29. Pan and seal for offset pour-flush latrine**

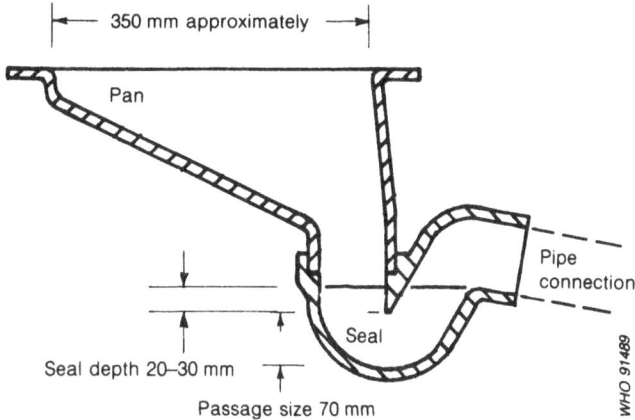

depends on the design of the pan or pedestal, the depth and volume of the water seal, and the minimum passage size through the seal. For a water seal directly above the pit about 1 litre of water is normally sufficient for flushing. Two litres may be required for an offset pit and a minimum of 3 litres for an improved pedestal pan and offset pit.

The depth of the water seal is measured as the depth of water that would have to be removed from a fully filled trap to allow the passage of air (Fig. 7.28). The seal volume is the amount of water held within the trap when the unit is not being used, and the minimum passage size is the opening through which the water must flow and which may be of a smaller diameter than the connecting pipe. The depth of the seal in a conventional WC is approximately 50 mm. However, the deeper the seal the more water is required for flushing. In pour-flush latrines, the depth of the seal is normally reduced to the minimum compatible with maintaining the seal in hot weather. The seal volume will be reduced by evaporation, the water loss being proportional to the time between consecutive flushings and the degree of exposure to direct sunlight and air movement. A minimum seal depth of 20 mm is considered reasonable with an optimum passage size of 70 mm (Mara, 1985b).

Water seals that can be removed during the dry season to minimize water usage are not recommended. It is likely that the seal would not be replaced at the beginning of the wet season and therefore the latrine would not work effectively.

## Types of water seal

Where the water seal services a direct pit, the pan and the seal should be made as a single piece with a hemispherical bowl known as a "gooseneck" trap. This is designed to discharge into the centre of the pit and not against the pit lining where it might cause damage. These types of seal can easily be damaged by users trying to clear blockages with a rod where the thin cement of the seal is unsupported. As direct pits have become less popular because of emptying difficulties, the use of the gooseneck trap has also declined.

In many countries, the pan is made separately from the seal to facilitate manufacture and to give the installer greater freedom as to where the offset pit is located in relation to the pan. The normal system, which has an inclined outlet, is known as a P-trap, while the system with a vertical outlet is called an S-trap.

## Water-seal materials

Pans and water seals may be produced by manufacturers or by project staff to standard specifications in a variety of materials. Ceramics, such as white vitreous china or other glazed earthenware, have traditionally been used for pans and pedestals. However, such items may be expensive to purchase and require careful attention to packing if they are to be transported safely. They may also be heavy and require a strengthened slab for a direct pit. Particularly because of the problems of transport and handling, the use of plastics for pans and water seals is becoming more common. Glass-fibre pans and high-density poly-ethylene (HDPE) water seals are light and easily transportable, even by bicycle, and are often preferred by users, even when more expensive than the cement-based systems described below.

The cheapest pans and seals are made from cement mortar (10–30 mm thick) close to the point of sale or delivery. They can be produced on a large scale without factory facilities, and can be repaired easily when damaged. Such units are likely to be rougher than manufactured pans and seals, and a reaction between urine and the cement normally leads to some staining of the surface and some odour from the trap. This can be minimized by the addition of marble dust and chippings to the cement mortar. When dry, the surface can then be rubbed down with carborundum stones to provide an attractive mosaic finish. Colourings may also be added to the mortar to give a more attractive appearance.

An alternative method of production uses casting boards to cast the pan and seal in two halves with a 1:2:2 concrete mix pressed around the form. After 24 hours the two sections can be removed from the moulds and joined together with neat cement, the inner surface also being smoothed off with neat cement. One disadvantage of having the pan and water seal in one piece is that the trap cannot be rotated in the direction of the offset pit.

The Thai model, which is now in use in about 3 million rural homes, employs a two-part mould and is cast in a single step, including the platform, without the need for grouting pieces together. The depth and angle of the seal are uniform. Large numbers of moulds can be cast quickly, thus facilitating production of pans and seals so that large numbers of households can have pour-flush latrines in a very short period of time (J. T. Visscher, personal communication).

Making the pan and trap separately enables very simple forms to be used. These may be built up from clay and husk or plastered brick or concrete which can be reused many times. A release agent is needed to break the bond between the mould and the new concrete. Proprietary agents are available, though used engine oil or even cow-dung wash have proved to be cheap and effective.

Pedestals designed for pour-flushing with small quantities of water (about 3 litres) are normally made of ceramic to ensure a smooth finish. Less efficient units may be made using cement-based methods with ferrocement, fibre-reinforced cement and concrete with marble chippings.

## Pipes and junction chambers

The water seal may be connected to the offset pit by conventional pipework (see Fig. 6.9, p. 53) or by a covered drain (see Fig. 6.10, p. 54). Where double pits are in use, a junction chamber or inspection chamber (see Fig. 6.15, p. 56) is required whereby the flow can be directed into one pit or the other.

The pipe or channel should be not less than 75 mm wide and should be as smooth and direct as possible. Any roughness or sharp bends will tend to slow the passage of excreta, eventually leading to a build-up of deposits and a blockage. The cheapest available non-pressure pipes will be adequate, whether in fired clay, plastic or asbestos cement. The minimum slope should be 1 in 30 for smooth pipes and 1 in 15 for rougher pipes or hand-shaped channels. If the slope is too steep there is a danger of solids being deposited in the pipe.

Special care must be taken where the pipe passes through the superstructure wall (see Fig. 6.12 and 6.13, p. 55). If possible, some degree of flexibility is required at the pipe joints or in the channel so that differential settlement of the latrine superstructure or the pit lining will not cause damage. There is unlikely to be significant loading on the ground above the connecting pipe, but where there is any possibility of vehicles crossing the area between latrine and pit, conventional pipe-bedding and protection should be used.

The pipe or drain should extend some distance into the pit so that the wastewater discharges directly towards the centre and does not dribble down the pit walls, with a consequent build up of deposits.

Where a covered drain is used to connect a double-pit system, a simple Y-junction can be constructed to divert the flow. The junction in a pipework connection between pits and latrine requires a chamber which should be of sufficient size to allow for ease of construction of the concrete benching. It must also allow for the flow to be diverted from one pit to another with a temporary blockage in one or other arm of the Y-junction. A minimum internal dimension of 250 mm is recommended (Roy et al., 1984). The chamber cover slab needs to be removable to allow for access to divert the flow, but also has to be heavy enough and fixed in such a way that it is difficult for children to remove.

## Vent pipes

**Fig. 7.30. Straight vent pipe**

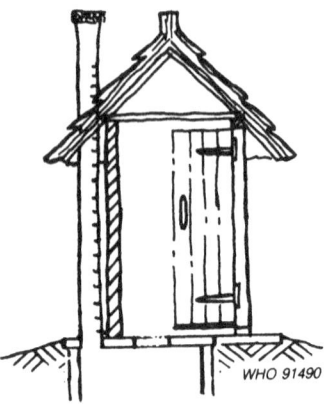

WHO 91490

The vent pipe, i.e., the tube connecting the latrine pit to the open air above the pit, serves two purposes: (1) to create a draught of air from the superstructure, through the squat hole and out of the pit, passing up the vent; (2) to act as a light source which will attract flies to the screen trap which is attached to the top of the vent. Normally the vent pipe is straight and rises vertically above the pit so that the daylight at the top can be seen directly by any flies in the pit (Fig. 7.30). A straight pipe also maximizes the air flow; bends in the vent absorb part of the energy in the air movement.

With certain types of slab, or where existing slabs require upgrading with a vent, there may be a need to bring the pipe out horizontally underneath the slab before turning to the vertical. In this situation an ancillary light source is required in the form of a glass or perspex window at the bend (Fig. 7.31). Flies in the pit are first attracted to the light source at the window. They cannot escape from the vent at that point so, following the air flow upwards, they then go towards the light at the top of the vent.

**Fig. 7.31. Angled vent pipe with window**

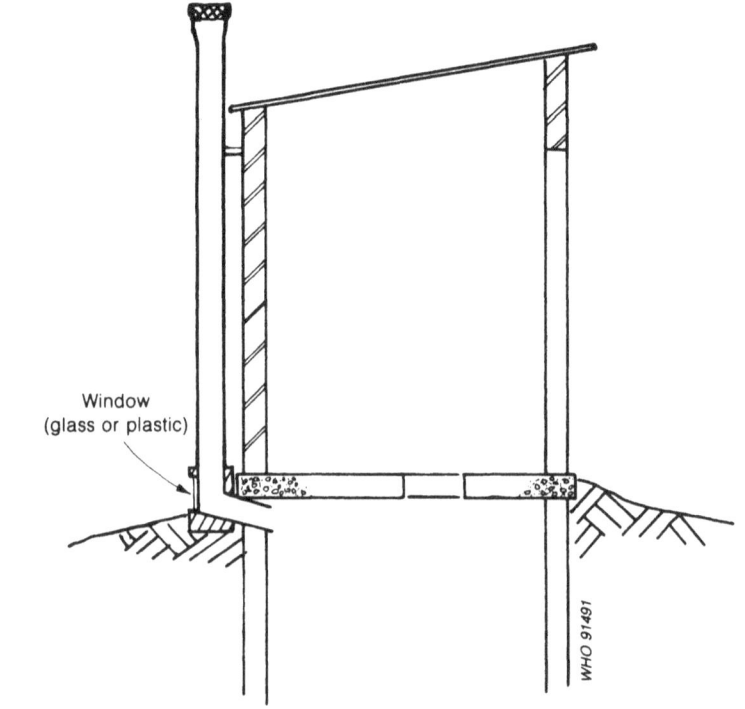

Window (glass or plastic)

WHO 91491

116

The draught through the vent is created primarily by the movement of wind across the top of the pipe. This air movement creates a suction effect, sucking air out of the pit and up the vent. To achieve satisfactory air movement, the top of the vent should be at least 500 mm above the highest part of the roof, except where the roof is conical, in which case the pipe should reach at least the height of the roof apex. However, if the pipe can be extended even higher, a stronger updraught will be created in the vent. Wind speed increases even at slightly higher elevations above the ground, which creates a stronger suction effect. Also, the higher the vent, the less likely it is to be shielded by buildings or other obstructions which may cause air turbulence and reduce or even reverse the updraught in the vent. Any large trees or overhanging branches close to the vent may significantly affect air movement and thus reduce the effectiveness of the ventilated latrine. Similarly, a rain cowl should not be placed on top of the vent, as it will reduce the air flow; the amount of rain entering the pit is not likely to be significant.

The vent should therefore be located in the best position to catch any air movements across the upper end of the pipe. Vent pipes are normally placed outside the superstructure, particularly where the building materials available make it difficult to construct a watertight joint where the pipe would pass through the roof. Free-standing pipes may be secured to the wall of the superstructure using standard pipe fittings, strips of galvanized steel, galvanized wire or other non-corrosive material. Where possible, the vent should be located on the side of the building which faces the equator, that is the side which receives most sunlight. The warming of the surface of the vent pipe, raises the temperature of the air in the pipe, increasing the upward draught. Painting the vent black aids this thermal effect. However, the air movement over the top of the vent is the most significant factor in causing updraught and a vent placed inside the building will still work effectively.

The updraught may also be increased by using a spiral design for the superstructure, which funnels the air into the structure. If there are no other ventilation holes, this produces a positive pressure inside the structure, thus forcing air through the squat hole and the pit and up the vent. However, where the winds are particularly variable and often blow from a direction away from the superstructure opening, a negative pressure may be created which will suck foul air out of the pit and into the building (Fig. 7.32).

## Dimensions of the vent pipe

Vents may be square or round and can be constructed from a wide variety of materials. Circular vent pipes should normally have an internal diameter of at least 150 mm for smooth materials (PVC or asbestos cement) or 230 mm for rough surfaces (such as locally produced cement-rendered pipes), although in exposed places with high

**Fig. 7.32. Layouts for superstructures, vent pipes and pits**

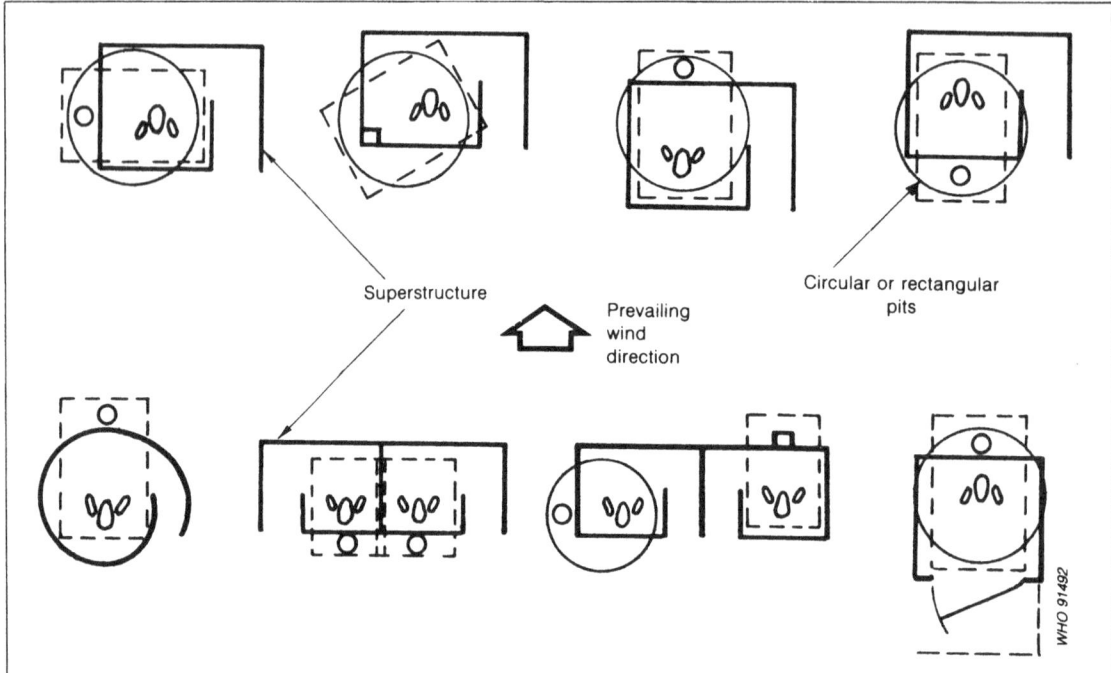

Superstructure

Prevailing wind direction

Circular or rectangular pits

WHO 91492

**Fig. 7.33. Belled vent with fly screen**

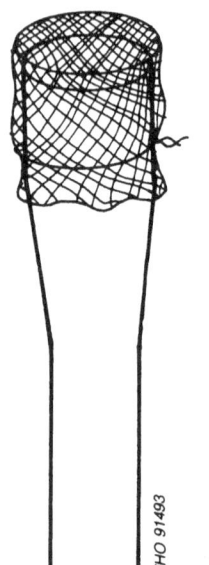

WHO 91493

wind speeds a smaller diameter may be sufficient. It is normally advantageous to enlarge the top of the vent pipe by about 50 mm to account for the head losses, that is, the reduction in energy and therefore in updraught caused by the air passing through the fine mesh of the flyscreen (Fig. 7.33). There is a danger that cobwebs, dirt or insect matter may build up on the screen, restricting air flow. Belling the top of the pipe can serve to balance these restrictions.

## Materials

Materials suitable for vent pipes include asbestos cement, unplasticized PVC, bricks, blocks, hollowed-out bamboo, ant-hill soil, cement-rendered reeds or bamboo, and cement-rendered hessian (Ryan & Mara, 1983). The choice of material will need to take into account durability, availability of materials and skills, cost, and availability of funds. Ordinary PVC becomes brittle when exposed to strong sunlight, so material with a special stabilizer should be used if possible. Because galvanized steel corrodes in a humid atmosphere, the use of thin sheets is not recommended for vent pipes except in very dry climates.

### Brick and block chimneys

Vent pipes may be made from bricks or blocks with cement mortar joints in the form of a chimney that is at least 230 mm$^2$ internally. The flyproof screen should be stretched over the top surface of the highest bricks. If it is built into the course joint one brick down, a receptacle is created which catches leaves and other debris. The chimney may be free-standing or built into the corner of the superstructure. Morgan & Mara (1982) suggested that thermal updraught in such chimneys continues well into the night because the brickwork retains heat which is released slowly to the air over a period of several hours.

### Locally made vent pipes

Reeds, poles, thin bamboo or strips of 10–20 mm of large bamboo can be tied together with wire or string to make a mat which forms a base for cement mortar. The mat, about 2.5 × 1.0 m, is rolled round rings made of green sticks to form a tube about 300 mm in diameter. Flyproof netting is fixed over one end of the tube, which is then laid on the ground. The upper part of the pipe is covered with a layer of cement mortar made with one part of cement to three parts of sand. When the mortar has dried the tube is put in position with the mortared part against the wall of the latrine. Then the outer part of the pipe is plastered with cement mortar. Alternatively the pipe may be rotated on the ground and completely plastered before erection.

A vent pipe can also be made with hessian. First, a 250-mm-diameter tube is formed of spot-welded steel mesh made of 4-mm bars at 100-mm centres (100 mm apart, centre to centre). Hessian or jute cloth is stitched tightly round the outside of the tube and flyproof netting is stitched over one end. Cement mortar, made of one part of cement to two parts of sand, is then brushed over the tube in several layers until a total thickness of about 10 mm is formed. The vent pipe is then fixed in place. Alternatively, a pipe may be made from ferrocement with three or four layers of mesh plastered with cement mortar and without any hessian.

### Fly screens

Fly screens should be made of material that will not be affected by temperature, sunlight, or the corrosive gases that are vented from the pit. Stainless steel or aluminium are considered to be best. Their comparatively high cost may be justified by their long life, especially as the screen accounts for a very small proportion of the total cost of the latrine. PVC-coated glass-fibre netting is relatively cheap and has lasted for more than seven years in Zimbabwe (Morgan & Mara, 1982). However, it tends to become brittle after about five years and is likely to tear at the point where it passes over the edge of the pipe. Ordinary plastic screens deteriorate quickly in sunlight. Painted mild steel mesh, commonly sold as window screening against mosquitos, and galvanized mild steel mesh last only a few months before corrosion by the pit gases renders them ineffective. Gases and sunlight weaken the screens but the actual tearing of the material is assumed to be caused by birds alighting or possibly by lizards which frequent the top of rough-walled vent pipes or simply by the tension within the flexing screen (P. R. Morgan, personal communication).

A mesh size of 1.2–1.5 mm is recommended. If the apertures are larger small flies can pass through. If the apertures are smaller there is too much resistance to the updraught of air. The screen should be firmly fixed to the top of the pipe. Netting may be fitted over the top of brick and block chimneys during building and on locally made vent pipes during fabrication. Screens may be glued to PVC pipes with epoxy resin or tied on with a piece of wire. Where there is a particular problem with mosquitos breeding in wet pits, it may be necessary to install removable traps over the squat hole or pedestal (Curtis & Hawkins, 1982).

Netting should be inspected regularly (at least once a year) to ensure that it is still in place and that it remains in good condition. Part of routine maintenance is to pour a bucketful of water through the screen and down the pipe to wash away cobwebs and other material.

## Superstructure

The building or superstructure of any latrine is required to give privacy and protection to the user. From the health point of view the superstructure is less important than the pit and slab. However, as most people initially desire sanitation because of the convenience and privacy of having their own facilities, it is important that the superstructure meets the users' needs. Many sanitation projects leave the design and construction of the superstructure to the user. Although there may be some benefit in having a uniform design, it is advantageous to involve the owner or user in the construction. A properly built superstructure should conform to certain guidelines, the most important of which are outlined below.

### Size

The size of the building should be such that people are encouraged to use the facility properly, without its becoming an oversized status symbol. If the floor area is much larger than the pit slab, people may be tempted to defecate on the floor, particularly if the squat hole has been fouled by previous users. The height should accommodate a person standing upright without his or her feeling oppressed by the roof. However, if people are used to stooping when going into buildings, a lower entrance may be acceptable or even preferred. Where latrines are also being used as wash rooms or bath houses, a larger area should be allowed for.

## Shape

Where the superstructure is not attached to the dwelling, there are two possible basic shapes (see Fig. 7.32): (1) a simple round or rectangular box, with or without a privacy wall; (2) a spiral, which may be round or rectangular. Although the spiral design uses more wall materials (while saving on the possibly more expensive door and hinges), it has the advantage of keeping the inside of the building partially dark and is therefore more suitable for ventilated pit latrines.

If there is a door in a spiral design the functioning of the latrine is not affected by its being left open. The design automatically incorporates a privacy screen. However, if the pit has only a short life and the superstructure will need to be moved to a new location when the pit is full, then a simpler structure may be more suitable.

In some cultures there may be a prohibition on facing in a particular direction when defecating. This must obviously be taken into account when the latrine is being positioned.

## Location

The latrine may be built as a free-standing unit within the compound or may be attached to the house. If it is reached from inside the house there is a greater likelihood that it will be properly maintained. It also has the advantage that access can be controlled more easily by the householder. However, greater care has to be taken of the pit lining because of its proximity to the house foundations and the pit must be accessible from outside the house for emptying. Offset pour-flush latrines have the advantage that the pit or pits may be sited in any convenient space, even in the most cramped urban conditions. The pits may even be under the footpath access to the latrine.

## Ventilation

It is desirable to provide openings in the superstructure or around the door to ensure adequate ventilation of the latrine. The inlet vents are most effective when they face the prevailing wind and should preferably be at a different height from the outlet vents to improve the efficiency of air change (Fig. 7.34). A minimum requirement of about six complete air changes per hour (10 m$^3$/hour) has been recommended by Ryan & Mara (1983). An opening of at least 0.15 m$^2$ should be adequate in most climates.

With a ventilated pit, the air movement is required to clear the superstructure of stale air by passing into the pit for exhaust through the vent pipe. Where there is a fairly constant prevailing wind, any openings should be on one side of the structure only, facing the wind, so

121

**Fig. 7.34. Ventilation in a pour-flush latrine**

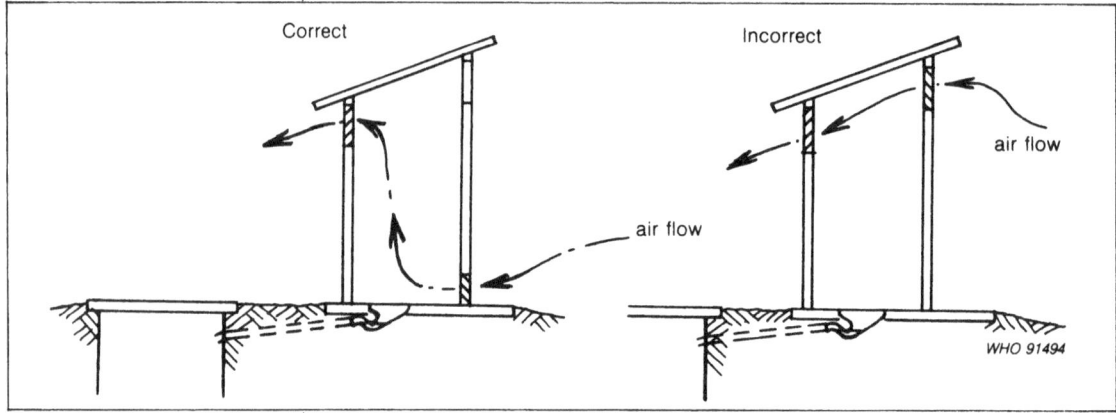

**Fig. 7.35. Ventilation in a VIP latrine**

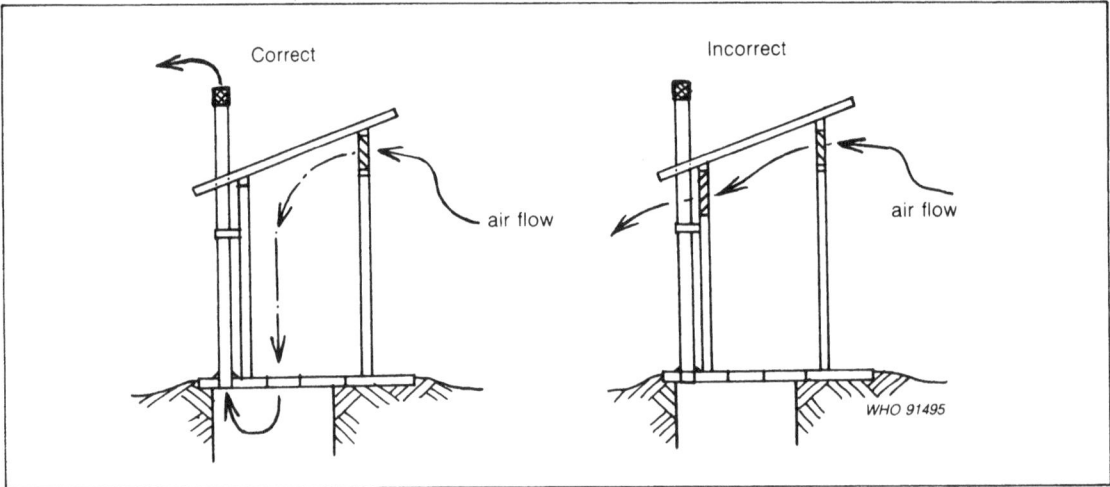

that there is no through draught and to ensure maximum air movement through the pit (Fig. 7.35). However, where the prevailing wind is variable, it may be necessary to have other openings in the superstructure to prevent a suction effect when the wind blows from a different direction. This can lead to foul air being sucked out of the pit through the superstructure, to the discomfort of the users.

The superstructure must be strong enough to support a vent pipe extending 500 mm above the roof line. Alternatively it may be found that a block or brick vent adds rigidity to the superstructure.

## Lighting

In general a latrine that is bright and light is more attractive to its users. A ventilated pit requires a partially darkened superstructure so that any flies in the pit are attracted by the daylight at the top of the vent pipe rather than light from the inside of the latrine. However, the internal walls of the superstructure may be whitewashed and some light allowed through ventilation openings.

Where possible, the opening spiral or door of a ventilated pit latrine should not face east or west as the low sun in the morning or evening would light up the inside of the structure and encourage the movement of flies out of the pit.

## Access

Contrary to normal building practice, the door is usually designed to open outwards to increase the usable space inside the building and to avoid hitting any footrests. This may not be practicable in grass-roofed structures with low eaves. In some cultures a privacy wall is required to screen the door. If a spiral design is used, no door is required (though one may be fitted if desired), which is an advantage where wood and other material for making doors are expensive or in short supply.

## Cleanliness

A superstructure that is left dirty and in a constant state of disrepair will soon be unused as a latrine and abandoned. It is therefore important that the building can be cleaned and maintained easily.

## Materials

The design of the superstructure and the materials employed normally depend upon the style and construction methods of other buildings in the area. It is to be expected that people will build their latrine out of the same materials as their dwelling—although perhaps to a slightly lower standard. The temptation for projects to produce structures in a grand style should be avoided. If the latrine buildings promoted by a project are of more expensive construction than local housing (even if they are temporarily subsidized) they cost more than people can ordinarily afford. This acts as a disincentive for new households to construct sanitation systems when the initial promotion is finished. Similarly, the introduction of new materials and methods should normally be avoided in a latrine programme as this diverts attention from the real purpose of the sanitation system. It is better to use local skills and materials which local tradesmen understand how to use and, most importantly, how to maintain.

Many different types of materials can be used and the most common of these are described below.

**Fig. 7.36. Privacy screens made from cheap locally available materials**

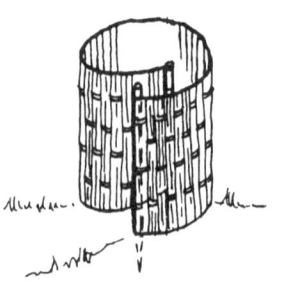

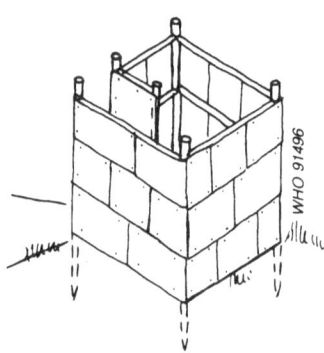

## Screens and fences

The superstructure does not necessarily have to be a roofed building, although there are obvious advantages in providing protection from the rain and sun. However, in some cultures people have become used to defecating in the open and find it objectionable to have to go into a small building. Also, where funds are limited the overall cost of the latrine is considerably reduced by erecting a simple fence made out of the cheapest locally available "waste" materials (such as grass, grain stalk, woven palm) to meet the need for privacy (Fig. 7.36).

In periurban areas, agricultural byproducts may not be available. Other waste products such as cardboard or beaten tin cans or sacking suspended on poles can provide the required privacy at very little cost.

It should be noted that a ventilated pit design needs a roofed and darkened superstructure.

## Mud and wattle

In many parts of the world the housing consists of mud and wattle, that is upright poles, with the bark removed, interwoven with small branches, the whole being plastered with mud. Such a system can be readily adapted to the needs of a small latrine, whether round or spiral, with a thatched roof made from palm leaves or grass thatch. Mud and wattle may be improved by nailing bamboo strips to straight upright

**Fig. 7.37. Reinforced mud and wattle superstructure**

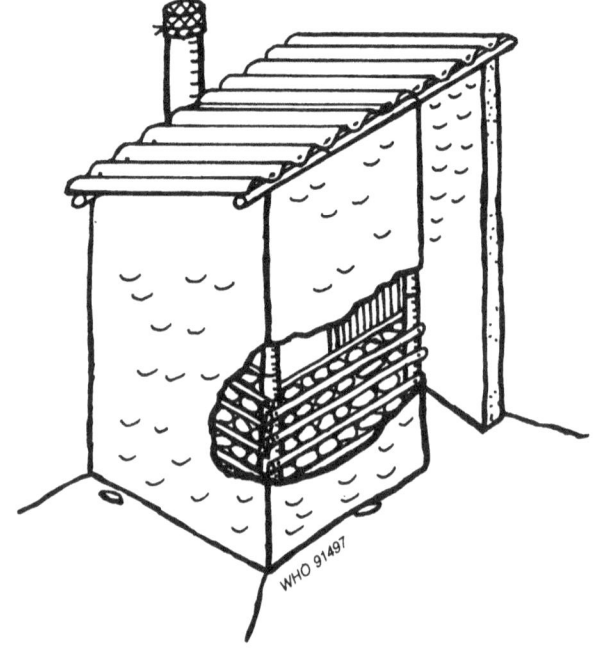

poles and filling the gaps with small stones before plastering with mud. A more regular, longer-lasting structure is obtained. This can be roofed with thatch or with beaten tin or even galvanized corrugated iron to provide a strong weatherproof structure (Fig. 7.37).

### Bamboo

Shelters can be made from larger-diameter bamboo poles forming the main frame with smaller bamboos nailed or strapped to them to form the walls. Alternatively palm leaves or bamboo matting can be used to fill in the walls of the bamboo frame.

### Sawn timber

Increasingly, sawn timber is becoming an expensive and rare commodity in low-income areas, but if off-cuts are available from a saw mill, these can be used to clad a simple timber-framed structure.

### Sun-dried bricks

Known as adobe, modagadol, kacha or by other local names, these bricks are simply made from a mixture of well-puddled and tempered clay. Moulded in simple wooden formers, they are allowed to dry slowly, out of direct sunlight. They can be strengthened with the addition of natural fibres such as fine grasses or coconut fibres. The superstructure is erected slowly using mud mortar, and where necessary the walls can be strengthened with the addition of fencing wire on alternate horizontal joints. Care must be taken to ensure that the walls are not made too thick if the superstructure is built above a pit. A great weight of walling can exert undue pressure on the foundations and sides of the pit and may lead to collapse.

### Machine-pressed blocks

This technique employs a portable steel press to compact prepared soils in order to produce regular blocks. The blocks may be stabilized with up to 8% of cement or lime depending upon the character of the soils used and the degree of exposure of the finished wall. The blocks are laid in mud mortar and can be plastered externally with mud mortar which requires attention every couple of wet seasons. However, as is the case with the sun-dried bricks, care has to be taken to ensure that walls are not made too thick and heavy.

### Fired bricks

Where also used for housing, these make an excellent material for latrine construction. To exert minimum pressure on the ground, a half-brick wall (112 mm thick) built in cement mortar is used with pillars at the corners. If mud is used as the mortar to reduce costs then a one-brick wall (225 mm thick) should be constructed.

### Concrete blocks

Where a more expensive standard is acceptable, or if firewood for brick firing is restricted, concrete blocks can be made by hand on site or purchased from a local manufacturer. The blocks are usually 150 mm thick but to reduce materials 65-mm blocks can be made. However, greater skill is required in the laying of these blocks and it is unlikely that a householder would be able to build without skilled assistance.

### Stone

Traditional building techniques with stones are sometimes used for latrine construction. This is normally to be avoided over direct pits as the thickness of the walls (often 450 mm or more) exerts a high load, requiring a strong pit lining for support. Stone buildings are quite acceptable, however, for offset pits.

### Ferrocement

A strong cement mortar pressed into three or four layers of wire mesh forms a strong, reasonably stiff membrane known as ferrocement. This material has been used successfully for spiral superstructures but can only be used where cement costs are low and the people are willing to accept a new technology along with their new latrines.

### Other materials

Plasticized materials, corrugated asbestos cement, galvanized iron and aluminium sheets are also used.

## Roofing

Materials such as thatch, palm leaves, clay tiles, fibre-cement tiles, wood shingles, corrugated iron, corrugated aluminium, asbestos cement, ferrocement and precast concrete can all be used for roofing the latrine superstructure. An important point to note is that the roof must be adequately tied into the wall structure and the walls must be strong enough to resist the uplift of high winds. Some materials, for example, galvanized corrugated iron, lead to greatly increased temperatures inside the latrine which may increase odour and make the building less pleasant to use.

## Doors

A door is not required for efficient functioning of most latrines. However, for various reasons, users often wish to have a sawn timber door. Where possible it is advisable to mount the door on self-closing hinges. Doors can also be made from beaten tins or corrugated iron on a wooden frame, bamboo strips or anything else that is available. Simple curtains may suffice where timber is scarce. A door is not necessarily required for privacy of the user. Where spiral designs have become common it is normal for people to knock on the outside of the structure before entering to warn anybody using the latrine of their approach.

Hinges do not have to be manufactured in steel; strips of old car tyres or leather from old shoes can equally well be used.

## Conclusion

In conclusion it may be emphasized that a superstructure is usually required first for privacy and secondly as a shelter for the user from the wind and rain. Brandberg (1985) asked the question, "Why should a latrine look like a house?" to demonstrate that the poorest people need not be excluded from the benefits of sanitation because they cannot afford the superstructure. A simple screen for privacy can adequately serve as a first phase while funds are found for a building. At a later stage materials in common use for house construction in the area will be suitable for building the latrine superstructure.

CHAPTER 8
# Design examples

## Introduction

The design of a latrine is governed by both consumer expectations and public health requirements. Although basic design factors remain the same (pit volume, septic tank retention time, etc.), the factors that govern the final cost of the latrine are controlled by local circumstances and requirements.

It is not feasible to illustrate all the possible design options. However, this chapter gives details of how to determine the basic dimensions for the most common designs and gives examples to illustrate the design procedure.

## Pit latrine design

### Pit size

When calculating the dimensions of a hole for a pit latrine, three conditions must be satisfied.

1. The pit should have sufficient storage capacity for all the sludge that will accumulate during its operational life or before its planned emptying.
2. At the end of the pit's operational life there should still be sufficient space left for the contents to be covered with a sufficient depth of soil to prevent surface contamination with pathogenic organisms (soil seal depth).
3. There should be sufficient wall area available at all times to enable any liquid in the pit to infiltrate the surrounding soil.

### *Storage volume*

The storage volume required to accommodate the sludge that accumulates in the pit during its operational life can be calculated from:

$$V = N \times P \times R$$

where $V$ = the effective volume of the pit (m³)
  $N$ = the effective life of the pit (years)
  $P$ = the average number of people who use the pit each day
  $R$ = the estimated sludge accumulation rate for a single person (m³ per year).

Once the effective volume of the pit has been calculated, the plan area is decided. This should be based on local preference, ground conditions and construction materials, and is generally circular or rectangular in shape. Note that only the area inside the lining is utilized for sludge accumulation, not the excavated area.

Having determined the plan shape and area, the depth of pit required for sludge accumulation is calculated as follows:

$$\text{Sludge depth} = \frac{\text{total sludge volume } (V)}{\text{plan area}}$$

### Soil seal depth

This is usually taken as 0.5 m. In the case of double pit latrines it is the depth to the bottom of the inlet drain.

### Infiltration area

In communities where people use water for anal cleaning or bathe in the toilet, a considerable amount of water may enter the pit. If it is assumed that the soil pores below the sludge surface are blocked, then additional wall area must be allowed for infiltration of the liquids above the sludge.

The infiltration area cannot include the soil seal depth since the top 0.5 m of a pit has a fully sealed lining.

Assuming that all the liquid entering the pit lies on top of the sludge, then the liquid depth will rise until the area of contact between liquid and soil is large enough to permit infiltration of the daily intake of liquid.

### Pit depth

The total depth of the pit is calculated as follows:

Pit depth = sludge depth + infiltration depth + soil seal depth

### ■ Example 8.1

*A family of six intends to dig a pit latrine with an operational life of 20 years. The family uses newspaper and corncobs for anal cleaning, and sullage is disposed of separately.*

■ *Sludge volume*
$$V = N \times P \times R$$

The values of $N$ and $P$ are given (20 years and 6 people) but the sludge accumulation rate $(R)$ is not. In the absence of local information the rate given in Chapter 5 can be used. The accumulation rate cannot be determined without some knowledge of the depth to the water table. Assuming this is greater than the likely pit depth, an accumulation rate of 90 l/year is used (see Table 5.3).

$$\text{Sludge volume} = 6 \times 20 \times \frac{90}{1000} \ (1 \text{ m}^3 = 1000 \text{ litres})$$

$$= 10.8 \text{ m}^3$$

If it is found that the pit does enter the groundwater, then the calculation should be done again using the appropriate sludge accumulation rate (60 l/year, from Table 5.3).

■ *Plan area*

The pit will be rectangular, with internal dimensions of 1.2 m by 2.0 m. Thus the depth required for sludge is:

$$\frac{10.8}{1.2 \times 2.0} = 4.5 \text{ m}$$

■ *Infiltration area*

Since solid objects are used for anal cleaning and sullage is disposed of elsewhere, there will be very little liquid to infiltrate. Accordingly the infiltration area can be ignored.

■ *Soil seal depth*

Assumed to be 0.5 m. Therefore the designed pit depth is:

$$4.5 + 0.5 \text{ m} = 5 \text{ m}.$$

This is very deep and consideration could be given to increasing the plan area or reducing the life of the pit.

■ **Example 8.2**

*A family of six intends to construct a pit latrine to last 20 years. The family uses water for anal cleaning and intends to use the toilet as a bathing area. The ground is mainly a fine sand with a water table 3 m below the surface.*

■ *Sludge volume*

Using the figures given in Table 5.3, the sludge accumulation rate will be 60 l/year above the water table and 40 l/year below. First assume that the pit will be mainly above the water table. If it is found that it enters into the groundwater by more than 1.0 m then the volume can be recalculated.

$$\text{Volume } (V) = N \times P \times R$$

$$= 6 \times 20 \times \frac{60}{1000}$$

$$= 7.2 \text{ m}^3$$

■ *Sludge depth*

If the pit is to be circular, with an inside diameter of 1.3 m, the sludge depth will be:

$$\frac{\text{Sludge volume}}{\text{Plan area}} = \frac{7.2 \times 4}{\pi \times 1.3^2}$$

$$= 5.42 \text{ m}$$

A pit of these dimensions would mean that most of the sludge would collect below the water table. Therefore the volume should be re-calculated using a sludge accumulation rate of 40 l/year.

$$V = 6 \times 20 \times 0.04$$

$$= 4.8 \text{ m}^3$$

Therefore the new sludge depth will be:

$$\frac{4.8 \times 4}{\pi \times 1.3^2} = 3.62 \text{ m}$$

■ *Infiltration rate*

The infiltration capacity of a fine sandy soil is about 33 l/m² per day (see Table 5.4). Assuming the volume of water entering the pit each day is 200 l then the infiltration area required will be:

$$\frac{200}{33} = 6.1 \text{ m}^2$$

Therefore liquid will build up in the pit until a contact area of 6.1 m² is achieved.

$$\text{Water depth} = \frac{\text{infiltration area}}{\text{pit circumference}}$$

$$= \frac{6.1}{\pi \times 1.3}$$

$$= 1.49 \text{ m}$$

Assuming a soil seal depth of 0.5 m, the total depth required for the pit is:

$$3.62 + 1.49 + 0.5 = 5.61 \text{ m}$$

This is a slight underestimate of the required depth because some of the sludge will accumulate above the groundwater level. Bearing in mind the inaccuracy of the basic design data, however, it is not necessary to carry out a more accurate calculation.

■ **Example 8.3**

*An offset pour-flush double-pit latrine is to be constructed for a family of six who use water for anal cleaning. The groundwater table is within 0.5 m of the surface during the rainy season and the soil is a sandy silt.*

■ *Sludge volume*
As for the previous examples:

$$V = N \times P \times R$$

In a large pit the value of $R$ would be taken as 40 l/year (see Table 5.3) but as this is a double pit, full consolidation of the sludge is unlikely to have taken place within the time taken to fill the pit (generally 2 years). Therefore a higher sludge accumulation rate (such as 60 l/year) should be used.

$$\text{Sludge volume} = 6 \times 2 \times \frac{60}{1000}$$

$$= 0.72 \text{ m}^3$$

■ *Sludge depth*
If each pit is 1.2 m wide and 1.2 m long, the sludge depth will be:

$$\frac{0.72}{1.2 \times 1.2} = 0.5 \text{ m}$$

■ *Infiltration depth*
An offset pour-flush toilet uses about 3 l of water per flush. Assuming 20 flushes per day the total liquid inflow will be:

$$3 \times 20 = 60 \text{ litres}$$

If 6 l of urine enter the pit each day, the total daily inflow of liquid will be 66 l. The infiltration rate for sandy silt is about 25 l/m² per day (see Table 5.4); therefore the infiltration area required is:

$$\frac{66}{25} = 2.6 \text{ m}^2$$

The perimeter length of each pit is $1.2 \times 4 = 4.8$ m, therefore the liquid depth will be:

$$\frac{2.6}{4.8} = 0.5 \text{ m}$$

■ *Pit depth*
The pit depth is the sum of the component depths, i.e.:

| | |
|---|---|
| depth to bottom of inlet pipe | 0.2 m |
| liquid depth | 0.5 m |
| sludge thickness | 0.5 m |
| | |
| Total depth of each pit below ground level | 1.2 m |

## Septic tank design

### ■ *Example 8.4*

*Design a septic tank suitable for a household with up to eight occupants in a low-density housing area in which the houses have full plumbing, all household wastes go to the septic tank and the nominal water supply is 200 l per person per day. Water is used for anal cleaning and the ambient temperature is not less than 25°C for most of the year.*

### ■ *Stage 1*
Volume of liquid entering the tank each day

$$A = P \times q$$

where $A$ = volume of liquid to be stored in the septic tank
$P$ = number of people using the tank
$q$ = sewage flow = 90% of the daily water consumption per person ($Q$).

$$q = 0.9 \times Q = 0.9 \times 200$$

$$= 180 \text{ litres per person per day.}$$

Therefore $\qquad A = 8 \times 180 = 1440 \text{ litres}$

### ■ *Stage 2*
The volume of sludge and scum is given by

$$B = P \times N \times F \times S$$

where $B$ = volume of sludge and scum
$P$ = number of people using the tank
$N$ = period between desludgings
$F$ = sizing factor (see Table 6.2)
$S$ = sludge and scum accumulation rate (see Chapter 6)

Assume $N$ is 3 years; from Table 6.2, $F = 1.0$; as all wastes go to septic tank $S = 40$ l per person per year.
Therefore:

$$B = 8 \times 3 \times 1.0 \times 40$$

$$= 960 \text{ litres}$$

### ■ *Stage 3*

$$\text{Total tank volume} = A + B$$

$$= 1440 + 960$$

$$= 2400 \text{ litres } (2.4 \text{ m}^3)$$

### ■ *Stage 4*
Assume liquid depth = 1.5 m
Assume tank width is $W$ m

**Fig. 8.1. Internal dimensions of the septic tank designed in example 8.4**

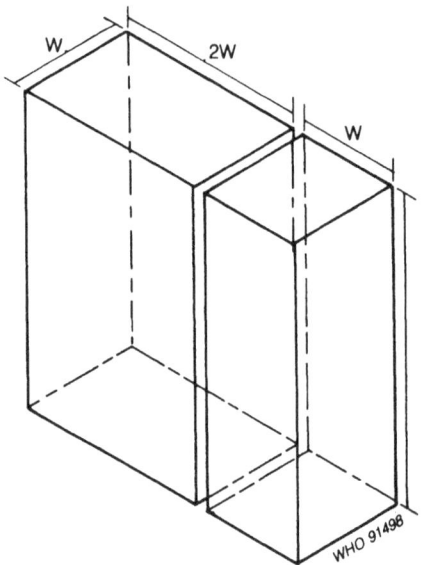

Assume two compartments, length of first $= 2W$
length of second $= W$

This tank is illustrated in Fig. 8.1.

Volume of tank $(V) = 1.5 \times (2W + W) \times W$
$$= 4.5W^2$$
Thus $4.5\,W^2 = 2.4\,\text{m}^3$
$$W = 0.73$$

Therefore:
width of tank                           $= 0.73\,\text{m}$
length of first compartment    $= 1.46\,\text{m}$
length of second compartment  $= 0.73\,\text{m}$
Depth of tank from floor to soffit of cover slab

$$= \text{liquid depth} + \text{freeboard}$$
$$= 1.5 + 0.3$$
$$= 1.8\,\text{m}$$

## Flotation

Since septic tanks have sealed walls and floor, the design must be checked to make sure that the tank does not float out of the ground. Flotation will occur if the total mass of the empty septic tank is less than the mass of the water it displaces. This will only happen if the groundwater level is higher than the bottom of the tank.

Calculate the mass of the walls, floor, roof and any baffle walls (concrete: 2400 kg/m³; brickwork: 1500 kg/m³). Measure the volume of the tank (outside dimensions) between the highest groundwater level and the bottom of the tank. Multiply the volume by the density of water (1000 kg/m³). This gives the mass of water displaced.

If the mass of water displaced is greater than the total mass of the empty septic tank then the tank may float. This can be prevented by increasing the mass of the structure (e.g., by increasing the thickness of the floor or walls) or reducing the amount of the tank that is below the water table.

## Soil pressure

For large tanks, such as for a school or a number of houses, it is necessary to check that the side walls of the tank are not likely to collapse owing to the outside soil and water pressure. This is most likely when the tank is empty. Such a calculation is beyond the scope of this book, and reference should be made to a manual on reinforced concrete or masonry design.

### ■ *Example 8.5*

*Design a septic tank for a household having five occupants in a medium-density housing area in which the houses have full plumbing. Only WC wastes go to the septic tank, and paper is used for anal cleaning. The ambient temperature is more than 10°C throughout the year.*

### ■ *Stage 1*
Daily volume of liquid

$$A = P \times q$$

If the WC has a 10-litre cistern and each person flushes it four times a day, the sewage flow $q = 4 \times 10 = 40$ litres per person per day and $A = 5 \times 40 = 200$ litres.

### ■ *Stage 2*
Volume for sludge and scum

$$B = P \times N \times F \times S$$

Assume $N$ is 3 years; from Table 6.2, $F = 1.0$; as only WC wastes go to septic tank $S = 25$ litres per person per year.

So $$B = 5 \times 3 \times 1.0 \times 25$$

$$= 375 \text{ litres}$$

### ■ *Stage 3*
Total tank volume $V = A + B$

$$= 200 + 375$$

$$= 575 \text{ l } (0.575 \text{ m}^3)$$

As this is less than the minimum recommended volume of 1.0 m³, the dimensions for the minimum volume should be calculated.

■ *Stage 4*

Assume liquid depth = 1.5 m.
Assume tank width is $W$ m.
Assume two compartments:

length of first      = $2W$
length of second   = $W$
Volume of tank     = $1.5 \times (2W + W) \times W$

$$= 4.5\, W^2$$

If $4.5\, W^2 = 1.0$ m³,

then $W = 0.47$ m

As this is less than the recommended minimum width of 0.6 m, assume $W = 0.6$ m.

Length of first compartment $(2W) = 1.2$ m

Length of second compartment $(W) = 0.6$ m

Depth of tank from floor to soffit of cover slab

$$= 1.5 \text{ m (liquid depth)} + 0.3 \text{ m (freeboard)}$$

$$= 1.8 \text{ m}$$

The tank volume (excluding freeboard) is:

$$(1.2 + 0.6) \times 0.6 \times 1.5 = 1.62 \text{ m}^3$$

which is larger than the required volume calculated in stage 3. This is no disadvantage; in practice the minimum retention time will be greater than 24 hours or the tank will provide longer service than three years before requiring desludging.

## Aqua-privy design

Aqua-privies are basically small septic tanks. They have the same purpose as septic tanks and work in the same way. It is recommended therefore that they are designed in the same way as septic tanks. It is also recommended that the minimum size of tank should be 1.0 m³. This is because smaller tanks are more difficult to build and the turbulence produced by the inflow will prevent proper settlement.

## Disposal of effluent from septic tanks and aqua-privies

### ■ *Example 8.6*

*Determine the size of soakpit required in porous silty clay to dispose of the effluent from the septic tank considered in Example 8.5.*

From Example 8.5, the sewage flow is 200 litres per day.
From Table 5.4, the infiltration rate for sewage is 20 l per m² per day.

Therefore, the wall area required is $\dfrac{200}{20} = 10 \text{ m}^2$

If the pit is 1.5 m in diameter, then the depth required from the bottom of the pipe from the septic tank to the bottom of the pit is:

$$\frac{10}{\pi \times 1.5} = 2.12 \text{ m}$$

### ■ *Example 8.7*

*Determine the size of drainage field required in porous silty clay to dispose of the effluent from the septic tank considered in Example 8.4.*

From Example 8.4 the sewage flow is 1440 l per day.
From Table 5.4, the infiltration rate for sewage is 20 l per m² per day.
So the wall area required is $\dfrac{1440}{20} = 72 \text{ m}^2$

If the effective depth of the trench (the depth from the bottom of the pipe to the bottom of the trench) is 0.6 m, the length of trench required is:

$$\frac{72}{0.6 \times 2} = 60 \text{ m}$$

This allows for infiltration on both sides of the trench.

If the plot is large enough, the drainage field should consist of two trenches, each 30 m long, connected in series.

## Composting toilets

### Double-vault latrines

The design of a double-vault latrine is similar to that of a pit latrine, i.e., the volume of each vault is calculated using the formula:

$$V = N \times P \times R$$

where $V$ = the effective volume of the vault (m³)
$\quad\quad N$ = the number of years the vault must last before becoming full
$\quad\quad P$ = the average number of users
$\quad\quad R$ = the estimated sludge accumulation rate for a single person (m³ per year).

The difficulty with vault design is that very little information exists on the sludge accumulation rate in vaults where excreta are mixed with ash and other organic material, and there has been little research into the pathogen survival rate in such an environment.

### *Desludging period*

Pit latrines are usually designed such that excreta are not handled for two years. Since the inside of a composting toilet is similar to that of a pit latrine, it is reasonable to assume that it should be designed using similar parameters. However, some researchers disagree with this, saying that the low moisture content of the compost produces very alkaline conditions that destroy the pathogens in a much shorter time. Times as low as four months have been suggested. In the absence of more accurate information, however, a two-year retention time is recommended.

### Sludge accumulation rates

The accumulation rate for the excreta component of the compost can be determined in the same way as for a double-pit latrine. In the absence of more accurate local information, figures 50% greater than those given in Table 5.3 are suggested.

Estimating the volume of ash and other organic material is more difficult. Experience in Viet Nam indicates that approximately twice the volume of faeces has to be added (Jayaseelan et al., 1987). Rybczynski (1981) suggested five times the volume of faeces, and Kalbermattan et al. (1980) recommended allowing 0.3 m³ per person per year for all wastes.

In the absence of information to the contrary, it is suggested that the total sludge build-up rate is calculated as three times the estimated faecal build-up rate.

### ■ Example 8.8

*Design a double-vault composting toilet for a family of six who use paper for anal cleaning.*

The effective volume of each vault ($V$) must be:

$$2 \times 6 \times (0.06 \times 1.5 \times 3) = 3.24 \text{ m}^3$$

Vaults are usually sealed when they are three-quarters full, therefore the actual volume of the vault must be:

$$\frac{4}{3} \times 3.24 = 4.32 \text{ m}^3$$

If the vault has a plan area of $1.3 \times 1.3$ m, the depth will be:

$$\frac{4.32}{1.3 \times 1.3} = 2.56 \text{ m}$$

## Continuous composting toilets

Even fewer design data are available for continuous composting toilets than for double-vault latrines. Past designs have been empirical and little published information exists indicating the level of their success. It is suggested that, until more data are available, the size of the primary tank in the toilet should be based on the formulae and factors used for double-vault latrines. The second tank should be 10–20% of the size of the first tank. The floors of both tanks should slope at an angle of 30° to the horizontal. No design data exist for calculating the size and number of aeration channels or the diameter and height of the ventilation pipe.

### ■ *Example 8.9*

*Using the information given in Example 8.8, design an appropriate continuous composting toilet.*

From Example 8.8 the volume of the primary tank should be 4.32 m³.

The volume of the second tank will be:

$$4.3 \times 0.15 = 0.65 \text{ m}^3$$

Assuming the first tank is 1.2 m wide and 2.2 m long then its depth will be 1.65 m.

The length of the second tank will be: $\dfrac{0.65}{1.2 \times 1.65} = 0.33 \text{ m}$

This is short and would make emptying very difficult; increase the length to 0.5 m.

Since the vault floor must slope at an angle of 30°, the depth of excavation at the outlet end will be greater than the depth at the inlet.

Assuming the floor of the second tank is horizontal the internal floor level will be at a depth of:

$$1.65 + 2.2 \tan 30° = 2.9 \text{ m}$$

Fig. 8.2 shows the final internal dimensions of the tank.

**Fig. 8.2. Internal dimensions of the continuous composting toilet designed in example 8.9**

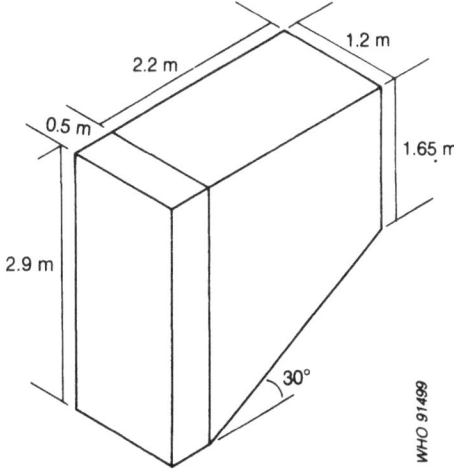

## PART III
# Planning and development of on-site sanitation projects

CHAPTER 9
# Planning

Many methods are used to provide or improve on-site sanitation. At one extreme, a project may involve detailed documentation (Grover, 1983) using the "project cycle" approach. At the other extreme, sanitation advances when individual householders build their own improved latrines, often because they have seen similar latrines built by neighbours. Many projects and programmes for improving sanitation lie between these extremes. Planning involves consideration of the local situation leading to selection of suitable types of sanitation. Designs are prepared and construction follows. On completion, and sometimes at intermediate stages, evaluation takes place.

With some projects, the form of planning and development is laid down by procedures which must be rigidly followed if external funds are to be released. However, in many successful programmes, development depends on the action of householders. Planning then leads to selection of appropriate forms of sanitation. Householders may be encouraged to adopt the selected types of sanitation by health education programmes, by technical or material support, or by other measures. The ways in which the different stages of planning and development may be regarded at various levels are shown in Table 9.1.

## The demand for sanitation

The initial demand for provision or improvement of sanitation in a particular area may come from the local people themselves or from a small group of active leaders in the community. Alternatively, the initiative may come from health officials, a government department, the organization responsible for water and sanitation, a bilateral aid agency, or a national or international voluntary organization. Ideally, sanitation improvements should be carried out in accordance with a national or regional sector plan and the adopted primary health care programme. A sector plan often covers both sanitation and water supply. It indicates the number of facilities to be provided, the number of people to be served in each district on a year-by-year basis during the planning period, and the resources needed. Particular attention is usually given to requirements for internal and external funding and to deficiencies in personnel of various categories.

There may be several reasons for a sanitation programme.

● There may be a genuine concern for health accompanied by an awareness that a high local level of disease is associated with existing sanitation practices.

## Table 9.1. The project cycle

| Government ministries and donor agencies | Implementing agency | Community |
|---|---|---|
| **Identification**<br>Definition of target population | | Felt need for improved sanitation |
| Determination of economic and health indicators, present service coverage and standards, objectives and policies, financial implications, staffing requirements, and training needs | | Exposure to health education |
| Assignment of planning responsibilities | | |
| **Pre-feasibility surveys**<br>Consideration of alternative projects to meet objectives taking into account technical, social, health, environmental, financial and economic criteria | Technical and social surveys<br><br>Planning with the community | Response to questions by health workers and government officials about health, wealth, water and sanitation |
| **Feasibility demonstration**<br>Detailed design and analysis of preferred/chosen project | Proving of recommended range of technologies at affordable price to satisfaction of representatives of proposed target group | Discussion regarding experimentation with affordable means of improving sanitation |
| **Appraisal and approval**<br>Independent check on planning, usually by representatives of funding source | | |
| Investment decision | | |
| Release of funds for project implementation | | |
| **Implementation**<br>*Consolidation* | Training, administrative support procedures, proving technology | Training of local people to assist with programme |
| | Determination of financial, material and technical support | Invitation to local artisans and contractors to participate |
| | | Drawings made available |

144

**Table 9.1. (Continued)**

| Government ministries and donor agencies | Implementing agency | Community |
|---|---|---|
| *Expansion* | | |
| | Mass promotion in the community | Publicity about the programme |
| | Health education, use of media | Systems available to copy |
| | Demonstration units as "sanitation supermarket" | Drawings made available |
| | Financial, material and technical assistance where appropriate | Financial assistance available |
| | | Local artisans and contractors available to help with building |
| | | Household decision as to purchase of sanitation system |
| *Operation and maintenance* | | |
| | Advice on responsibility of household to use and care for on-site system | Use of facilities |
| **Evaluation** | | |
| Identification of further projects | Identification of positive and negative aspects; reformulation of design criteria | Comments regarding desired improvements |

- Household latrines may be called for because of the convenience they offer to users.
- Good sanitation may be a status symbol.
- Existing excreta disposal methods may result in unacceptable pollution of surface water, soil or groundwater.
- Sometimes a demand for improved sanitation is associated with water supply. For example, a funding agency may require latrines to be constructed before it will provide piped water, or a water authority may wish to protect the catchment area for the supply to a nearby town by eliminating indiscriminate defecation. An increase in the amount of water provided to an area may lead to a demand for better wastewater disposal.

## Project definition

### Scope

Early in the planning process the extent of the programme or project must be assessed. This involves making an estimate of the number of people or households who will be covered. A house-by-house survey may be undertaken, or the necessary information obtained from health staff, government departments or local leaders.

## Priority areas

A list is drawn up comparing the needs of different areas. Priority should be given to people with especially poor facilities for excreta disposal and areas with a high incidence of diseases associated with poor sanitation. Areas with a high population density or congested housing may justify special attention. However, houses intended for temporary occupation may warrant less attention than permanent buildings.

Other factors that influence the selection of priority areas are the interest of the local communities in sanitation improvements and their record of participation in other projects. Ability and willingness to contribute financially may be other criteria for the selection of priority areas. Projects generally depend on a financial contribution from householders; occasionally priority is given to people most likely to pay or those willing to try new ideas. For projects that are externally funded, the poorest people may be selected for preferential treatment, on the assumption that better-off families should pay for their own latrines.

## Background information

Careful consideration should be given to all relevant factors in order to decide on the most appropriate form of sanitation and the most effective way of providing it. These factors include public health, socio-economic, cultural, financial, technological, institutional, and other considerations, as described on pages 148–154.

A large unified project may require several reports by agency officers or consultants. Long written reports are unnecessary for small projects and for programmes that consist of a succession of small schemes. However, whether a large or small scheme is planned, all relevant factors need to be carefully considered.

## The responsible agency

The planning and implementation of a simple programme for a few households may be within the capacity of a small committee of interested people, preferably with an enthusiastic leader. Larger pro-grammes may depend on government initiative, or on the support of an external body such as a bilateral agency, one of the international organizations, or a local nongovernmental organization. The degree of involvement of an agency varies considerably according to the nature of the project, the type of agency and other national and local conditions.

## Staff

Staff employed to plan sanitation projects should be carefully selected and prepared. Unless they have previously worked on similar programmes, the people appointed should receive formal or informal training, preferably on site with an existing sanitation project. It cannot be too strongly emphasized that the staff involved in all stages of a low-cost sanitation programme should be familiar with technological, management and sociological issues. They should also be familiar with the local financial and socioeconomic conditions, i.e., the standard of living of the local communities, and be aware of the important role that women, social workers and nongovernmental organizations can play.

## Community participation

The involvement of the community in any project is essential for its success, because almost all on-site sanitation work depends on decisions made by individual householders. The extent of involvement will vary in different countries. Urban communities often play a role that is quite different from that undertaken by village people, and this is likely to be different again from that of those living in dispersed family units. Some groups of people are homogeneous; others comprise various cultures and socioeconomic levels.

### Key leaders

Early contact should be made with key leaders, who may sometimes be identified with the assistance of the local health officials. The key leaders may be the chiefs and elders of villages, or people appointed by the government or political party. In some areas local schoolteachers or business people with education above the average may be useful as sources of local information and for an exchange of views.

### Minority groups

Whoever are selected as key leaders, care must be taken to ensure that the views of all sections of the community are represented. It may be necessary to seek out leaders of minority groups and representatives of those without political influence. In particular, the views and support of women should be sought. These are often best obtained by women social workers.

### Community needs and aspirations

Initial assumptions regarding the need for improved sanitation in the area as a whole and particularly in priority areas should be verified through contacts with key leaders and health workers. In particular, the incidence of excreta-related disease should be checked, as should awareness of relationships between sanitation and disease and of other disadvantages of existing excreta disposal practices, such as fly nuisance.

Care must be taken to avoid raising unreasonable expectations. At the same time, the local people should be made aware of the potential benefits of improved sanitation. When possible, even at the initial survey stage, key leaders should visit nearby completed projects to see good latrines in use. Simple drawings and models may also be used so that alternative technologies can be discussed.

Some idea of the readiness of the community to provide labour, money and materials for a latrine-construction programme should be obtained. Considerable skill is required to find out the true aspirations and priorities of the people. Answers to questions are often distorted because the interviewees wish to please the questioners. Small group discussions with minimum intervention by outsiders may be an effective means of finding out the true local opinion.

## Survey of the area

The most appropriate sanitation is that which best meets the needs and aspirations of the people within all local constraints. In order to assess what is most appropriate, a survey of the district should be carried out.

The survey may include both secondary and primary data. Secondary data are obtained from existing reports, maps and statistics. These should be critically examined and due allowance made for possible inaccuracy. For example, the information may not be up to date, or it may have been obtained from unreliable sources or collected hurriedly. Study of the available secondary data will reveal gaps that need to be filled by primary data.

Primary data are obtained by direct and indirect observation, measurement, household surveys, interviews and informal conversations. Care should be taken to ensure that those carrying out the survey have been properly trained. Any questionnaires used should be carefully planned to ensure that the answers reflect the true opinions of respondents.

A survey for a sanitation project may include the items listed below. In addition to information about the existing situation, any proposals for changes (and when they are likely to occur) should be noted.

### *Physical factors*

Of greatest importance is the local geology—the underlying rocks and the nature of the soil, in particular, how easy it is to dig and how stable the soil remains after excavation. It is also important to determine whether the soil is permeable so that water drains away, the depth of the top soil, how the soil varies with depth, the depth of hard rocks in which it is difficult to dig, and whether there are any fissures or boulders.

Natural gradients and the natural surface water drainage system should be noted, especially if there is much local variation. This may involve a study of the surface water hydrology and the climate, particularly the seasonal rainfall pattern. Areas that are subject to regular or occasional flooding should be noted. Any information that can be obtained about groundwater may also be useful, for example, the depth of the groundwater table, whether there is any seasonal variation or long-term change, the directions in which the groundwater flows, and its quality.

### Existing excreta disposal methods

It is essential to obtain as much information as possible about existing sanitation. A programme is usually intended to rectify an unsatisfactory situation and the extent of deficiency in sanitary provision is the baseline from which it starts. Any existing local sanitation that is satisfactory could give an indication of the most appropriate general solution. Improvements to existing systems are likely to be more acceptable than completely new ideas. In addition, examination of existing sanitation may provide useful technical information regarding such matters as soil infiltration capacity and rates of accumulation of solids.

Another advantage of obtaining accurate and complete information about existing sanitation is that it can contribute to the evaluation of the completed programme.

### Water supply

The service most closely related to sanitation is water supply, and careful note should be made of all water sources in the community. If possible, water sources should be visited and inspected. Claims by water authorities regarding the piped water supply service are often exaggerated, and the existence of water pipes and fittings should not be taken as evidence of satisfactory delivery of water. Pressure at the end of a long pipeline is often low, and the supply may be intermittent. Many people find it difficult to estimate distances in rural areas, so whenever possible the journey to collect water should be observed and timed.

Special care should be taken to check information relating to dependence on groundwater as a source of drinking-water. The depth of the water table and the location of wells and boreholes are particularly important because of the risk of pollution from pit latrines and soakpits. If possible, an analysis of the groundwater, including bacterial contamination and nitrate concentration, should be obtained. Comparison with analyses after the sanitation project has been implemented can then be used to monitor any groundwater pollution.

## Health and disease

The need for improved sanitation may be gauged from information about the prevalence of excreta-related diseases. Sometimes attendance records at local health centres yield this information, particularly in relation to diarrhoeal and parasitic diseases. However, the value of records depends upon the accuracy of diagnosis, the care with which records are kept, and the location of the health centre relative to the area served.

Data obtained in a health survey carried out before the start of a project may be compared with data from another survey after the project has been implemented as a means of assessing the effectiveness of improvements in sanitation. However, such baseline surveys are expensive and difficult to carry out successfully. They are normally only required where governments or donors require evidence of the efficacy of simple sanitation.

## Population and dwellings

Information obtained previously about the number of people and the number of houses to be served by the project should be checked and supplemented as necessary. Detailed demographic data, such as age and sex distribution may be significant, especially if it is customary for workers to move away from the area temporarily or permanently. Trends in any migration patterns should also be noted.

Aspects of housing that most affect sanitation are density, quality and level of occupancy. While low densities overall are usual in rural areas, it is not uncommon for dwellings in villages, and even in isolated family compounds, to be clustered at high density. The most relevant statistics are the open space belonging to each dwelling and the number of people occupying each dwelling. The quality of housing may indicate the economic level of the people and the efforts they are likely to put into improvements, including the construction of latrines. In many rural and periurban areas the majority of dwellings have been built by the occupants, who are therefore responsible for their own sanitation facilities. Improving the sanitation may be complicated where the occupant is not the owner, where a single dwelling is shared by several families, or where people occupy the upper storeys of multistorey buildings.

## Culture and traditions

Customs that influence the selection of the most appropriate type of latrine include:

- the preferred method of anal cleaning (water or solid material such as paper, leaves, stones, grass or corncobs);
- whether it is customary to defecate squatting or sitting;
- the degree of privacy favoured;

- the preferred location of latrines in relation to dwellings;
- any preference for bathing in the latrine after defecating;
- traditional use of human excreta or compost derived from human excreta as a fertilizer;
- objections to handling excreta, even when they have completely decomposed;
- any restriction regarding the use of the same defecation place by different groups, for example a taboo on use of the same place by men and women, adults and children, or even more specific categories such as fathers-in-law and daughters-in-law;
- any objections to the use of communal or family defecation places by certain people at certain times, such as women while menstruating.

### Communication and education

The ability and willingness of communities to accept new ideas, including new ideas about excreta disposal, are likely to be influenced by the extent of their outside contacts. In many places there is regular exchange of information through meeting people from other areas at markets, or when attending social functions. Literacy levels may determine the extent to which written or printed advice or instructions can be understood. It may be useful to find out how many members of the community own radios and television sets and whether they are in working order, and how many people read newspapers or see film shows, and in which languages. Understanding local terminology and traditional modes of communication, such as drama and song, may also be useful.

### Employment

While full information about employment of the local people is useful as background, of particular importance to sanitation planning is the location of workplaces. The practice of spending a high proportion of each day on farms that are distant from dwellings may influence the design of household sanitation. Similarly the extent of other activities away from home, such as attendance at markets or industrial employment, may point to a need to provide latrines at these places. Any seasonal variation in economic activity, income level, and location of workplace should be noted.

### The environment

Cleanliness of private dwellings and yards, and also of public roads, footpaths and open spaces, may give a good indication of the likely interest of communities in improving excreta disposal facilities. Methods commonly used for disposal of solid waste should be noted.

## Infrastructure

Ease of access by vehicles should also be checked, bearing in mind that many rural roads that are reasonably good in dry weather may be impassable for several weeks or months during the rainy season. Vehicular access to properties may affect the choice of type of latrine, for example, where full pits need to be emptied by vacuum tanker.

## Construction

While some householders may be able to build their own simple latrines, in many places construction will be undertaken by contractors or self-employed artisans. An assessment of the ability and reliability of local contractors and artisans is therefore required. The financial status of contractors may be relevant. Apart from latrine construction, firms or individuals may be able to prefabricate components, such as slabs, blocks, pans and pipes.

The availability and market price of materials and components likely to be used in the construction of latrines should be ascertained as accurately as possible. For material that can be obtained locally, such as sand and gravel, the actual cost of extraction and transport may be more relevant than market prices. Wage rates for skilled and unskilled labour should be noted.

## Availability of internal finance

An assessment should be made of the likely contribution that beneficiaries will make to the cost of latrine construction and maintenance. Money available in rural communities usually depends on the sale of agricultural produce and its seasonal variation; cash may only be available at harvest-time. In any community there may be income from wages and salaries, and from remittances received from absent members of families.

Attempts should be made to estimate willingness to spend money on sanitation, although it must be realized that statements made by individuals or community leaders regarding ability or willingness to pay are often unreliable. Responders usually answer questions in a way they think will give them greatest benefit. They may think that if they claim to be poorer than they are they will receive more outside help. Alternatively, they may exaggerate their ability to pay if they expect that this will ensure the implementation of outside-funded improvements.

Ability to pay may be based on the income of poorer sections of the community. In some places it has been found that payments for improved sanitation by the poorest people should not exceed 1% of their income, but up to 3% is acceptable for other economic groups (Kalbermatten et al., 1982).

### Availability of external finance

The fullest possible information should be obtained regarding grants, loans and subsidies likely to be available from local and central governments, bilateral donors, international and commercial banks, and other external sources.

## Comparison and selection of systems

Careful consideration should be given to all the technical factors described in Chapter 5 in order to select a number of appropriate types of latrine from those described in Chapters 4 and 6. A decision tree, like that shown in Fig. 9.1, may serve as a framework for selection. In effect, use of such an approach may eliminate some forms of sanitation, leaving others for further consideration.

Factors that are relevant in deciding whether a sanitation system that is technically feasible should be offered to householders and communities include the following:

- whether the system appears to be popular, as demonstrated by the number of householders who have already adopted it or by widespread interest in possessing it;
- the extent to which its use would fit in with local cultural and religious customs;
- the extent to which it would reduce pollution and health risks;
- the ease with which it can be provided by the people themselves, having regard to local skills and easily available materials;
- the cost, and particularly the cost of any materials, components and labour that cannot be provided by the householders;
- the ease with which it can be operated and maintained.

Having selected a number of options that are appropriate, the costs of each option can then be estimated. These should relate to a range of construction methods and materials. The total cost in both financial and economic terms of providing the required number of units for the project may then be calculated. Some agencies may favour least-cost solutions for externally funded projects, as discussed in Chapter 10.

When suitable options have been selected, the agency or the community itself must then go on to provide the latrines, giving each individual householder the maximum possible opportunity of choosing between alternative types, materials, finishes and other details. The stages in the implementation process are discussed in Chapter 11.

## Fig. 9.1. Decision tree for selection of sanitation

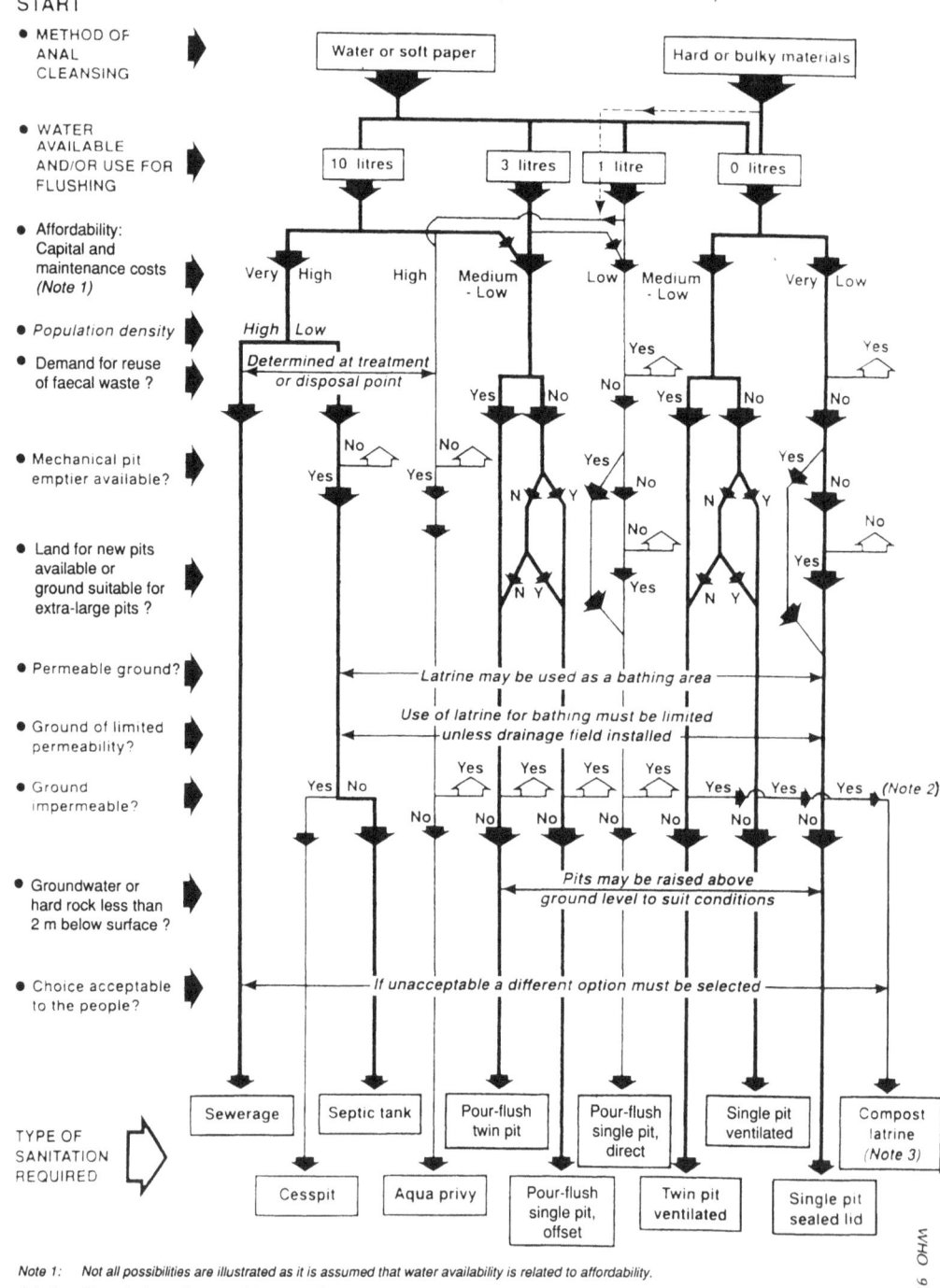

Note 1:   Not all possibilities are illustrated as it is assumed that water availability is related to affordability.

Note 2:   Use extra-large pits or consider composting.

Note 3:   Also dependent on willingness to collect urine separately, demand for compost, availability of ash or vegetable matter, etc.

WHO 91381

CHAPTER 10

# Institutional, economic and financial factors

## Institutional responsibilities

Any work on sanitation improvement is carried out within a framework of household, community and governmental relationships, all of which affect the manner in which a programme is executed. Of major importance are the organizations or institutions that have been given responsibility for or have an interest in some aspect of sanitation improvement. Such bodies may be governmental ministries, departments of ministries, urban municipalities, rural councils, nongovernmental agencies or recognized organizations.

In this book, a body outside the local community which takes primary responsibility for initiating, promoting, supervising or otherwise supporting a sanitation improvement project is generally referred to as an agency in order to distinguish it from other interested institutions. This agency may be a sectoral institution or a part of an institution. It may also be a special multidisciplinary team drawn from several institutions or even a nongovernmental organization working under the authority of a governmental institution.

### Projects or programmes

Improvements to sanitation practices involve projects and programmes. Projects are specific tasks with realizable goals within a specified time period. Programmes are continuous undertakings with long-term objectives. Protecting people and their environment from excreta-related disease and pollution is a continuous task which requires the responsible agency to take a long-term, programme approach.

Projects may be of vital importance to give a short-term boost to the sanitation programme and to enable people to make the next incremental improvement in their facilities. However, every project should be clearly related to existing sanitation programmes, with the relevant staff and institutions understanding its nature and objectives.

### Governmental involvement

#### *Allocation of responsibility*

Government ministries of health, water supply, rural development, local government, agriculture, and social welfare, and local government councils may all have an interest in sanitation. This concern may be at central, regional or local level. Ministries of finance and economic planning may also wish to exert some control. For a programme to succeed, there should be one lead agency, with a designated officer or management committee which has the responsibility and authority to take executive action.

### Integration of sectoral responsibilities

Nomination of a lead agency does not free other institutions from responsibility for a programme. Under their own terms of reference, they may want to play an active role in the promotion of sanitation, and may be able to provide specialist skills and inputs that are of vital importance. Consequently, it is necessary to define the responsibilities of all associated institutions, agencies and government officers at an early stage. The degree of involvement of any body will vary considerably according to the nature of the programme, the type of organization and other national and local conditions.

A forum or meeting for open discussion of needs and concerns may be of value. From this an intersectoral advisory committee can be drawn for more regular discussions of progress. However, it remains advisable to have a single lead agency responsible for decision-making rather than an intersectoral committee.

### Specialized sanitation support teams

Where a sanitation programme is being given a new impetus it is often found that the staff already have too many duties to be able to take on significant roles in a new project. Staff must either be released from other duties or new personnel appointed. The creation of a multidisciplinary "sanitation improvement team" may be an effective means of encouraging progress. However, the relation of such a team to the existing organizational structure should be defined, particularly with regard to its eventual re-absorption as part of the overall programme.

Specialized teams or agencies, where properly constituted, are often able to bypass the bureaucratic procedures and delays that exist in all institutions. Particularly where unconventional, community-based approaches are used, considerable flexibility is required from the facilitating agency. For example, staff may need to attend community meetings in the evenings or extension workers may need to make home visits when householders are home from work. Extra payment for overtime, or time off in exchange for late working, may have to be arranged.

### Flexibility within the institution and support team

As discussed in Chapter 11, there are considerable advantages in mobilizing the people, particularly with regard to the long-term sustainability of the improvements. However, in the short term there is no guarantee that the people will respond to the extent and at the rate desired by the agency.

The role of the agency may be made more difficult by non-acceptance of the preferred design standards, slow take-up of credits or materials, unfulfilled budgets, lengthy construction times and un-completed objectives. Particularly where outside donors are involved, there will be a pressure to produce measurable results. The agency has to organize its budgets and work plans in such a way that donors and any sponsoring institutions are able to understand what is happening and why, while retaining the flexibility required by the people.

### *Multilateral and nongovernmental organizations*

Many aid and development organizations become involved in sanitation programmes with the aim of improving the health of the people. Some may be based within the country, while others are externally supported. Some are able to draw on considerable experience over many years in different parts of the world, with funds and skilled personnel from different countries. Others have limited experience and/or funds but demonstrate a strong desire to assist the people. Their enthusiasm and ability to respond quickly to new ideas may be usefully harnessed for the good of the project.

The sponsoring institution has to decide how best to use all offers of help. The crucial task is to integrate the multilateral and nongovernmental organizations and the sectoral institutions, where appropriate, into the long-term programme, with the objective of limiting any tendency the smaller organizations may have to promote one-off projects that are not sustainable.

### Institution–householder linkage

To be effective, government institutions must have contacts with householders and the wider community that go beyond simply instructing the people what they must do. This is discussed more fully in Chapter 11. The lead agency should be constituted so that it can manage:

— community surveys, interviews, meetings, household visits;
— demonstration centres, sanitation "supermarkets", component purchase and/or production and sales;
— general or task-specific support staff, for example technical, social, financial and health staff;
— training of community members as facilitators;
— financial assistance; material assistance; technical assistance in construction;
— identification of contractors and skilled builders;

— standard specifications and target prices;
— ongoing support, in terms of technical assistance, and health education; and
— evaluation and monitoring.


## Human resources development

Human resources development includes the employment, supervision, continuing education and training, and occupational welfare of the people needed to do a job properly. The process should embrace planning, development of skills and training, and human resources management, with all aspects harmoniously geared to the achievement of specific goals.

Shortcomings in the preparation, implementation, operation and maintenance of sanitation schemes are often blamed on poor performance of programme staff and the ignorance of the people using the system. The usual response is to plan a training programme to educate all those involved in how to carry out their tasks correctly. However, such teaching may not in itself solve difficulties of performance. There are many factors to be considered in enabling people to perform to their full potential, and it is one of the roles of the programme manager to consider all aspects of human resources development.

Carefoot (1987) suggested that deficiencies in human performance, particularly with regard to water and sanitation activities, can generally be traced to one or more of the following: lack of skill or knowledge; environmental and/or management difficulties; or motivational, incentive or attitudinal causes. If lack of skills or knowledge is the primary cause of a problem, training is the likely solution. However, if problems stem from environmental and/or management causes, or from motivational causes, they will probably not be solved by training alone. In a number of surveys, managers involved with water and sanitation programmes have estimated that only 10–30% of performance difficulties are due to lack of skills or knowledge which can be rectified through training.

A "dual-focus" approach—on both the individual and the system within which the individual works—was therefore suggested by Carefoot in seeking solutions to performance problems. Development of skill should be complemented by the strengthening of the organizational environment, whether formal or informal, in which the person works.


## Programme participants

Before looking at the requirements for human resources development in more detail, the people who might need to be involved in a programme must be considered.

## Householders

One of the advantages of many on-site sanitation systems is that much of the work can be undertaken by the beneficiaries. Householders can plan, design and construct many elements of a latrine. Support is therefore required both for the individual householders and for the community to impart the necessary confidence that they can complete the task.

The special role of women in many countries in running the home, collecting water, and managing the sanitation system should not be underestimated. Many training programmes are automatically biased towards men or, by including men, exclude women. However, women have a vital part to play in the appropriate design, construction, operation and maintenance of excreta-disposal systems. Any human resources development programme must cater for the particular needs of women. Some programmes have also benefited from paying particular attention to the needs and role of children, both within formal education and informally in the community.

## Community leaders and councillors

Community leaders have their own special interests, particularly where communal decisions have to be made about some aspects of a sanitation scheme or where leaders can set an example to other householders.

## Artisans

In many projects there is a need for masons, bricklayers, drain-layers, carpenters, plumbers and other artisans to carry out part of the work. These workers often have experience in construction of houses and other buildings. Special skills may be required for the construction of latrines and associated works.

## Local contractors

Householders may require local contractors to carry out certain tasks for them, such as lining pits or constructing slabs. Where new techniques are being introduced or new forms of project support and funding used, contractors and subcontractors will require support.

## Programme and project staff

The numbers and categories of people needed to prepare and implement a project are largely determined by the nature and size of the project, type of agency, involvement of central and local government, whether the project forms part of an ongoing programme, and the degree to which the community participates.

Government health officers often play an essential part in sanitation improvement schemes, especially where the ministry of health is responsible for sanitation. Where a technical arm of government (such as a public works department) or an independent agency is responsible, management and supervision may be in the hands of technical officers. In some countries, health assistants, community and development officers and extension officers may be the link between an agency and the community. There is considerable variation in the terms used for different groups of workers and in the allocation of duties between these intermediate-level staff.

### Professional staff

Several kinds of professional staff may be concerned with sanitation improvement projects:

— public health engineers who are employed by an agency or by consultants working for an agency, with primary responsibility for the technical aspects of the programme;
— architects, planners, medical officers and development staff who, because of their jobs with agencies or government departments, are involved with the planning and implementation of sanitation;
— behavioural scientists, anthropologists, health staff, geologists, economists and others having specialist expertise that can be beneficially employed at some stage of planning or implementation; and
— administrators.

## Skills and knowledge training

If training is to be relevant and is to produce the desired results, it must be planned systematically. The objectives are to enhance people's breadth and depth of knowledge about their particular responsibilities, and to improve their ability to carry out particular tasks. In order to achieve these it is useful to follow a training cycle. This same cycle may be followed for householders as well as for professional engineers (Fig. 10.1).

### The training cycle

Preparation of any training programme begins with an assessment of training needs. This requires an organizational chart describing the different jobs to be carried out in order to complete the objective. The objective should not be limited to completion of initial construction but should also include operation and maintenance. Each of the jobs listed then requires a job description, that is, a detailed list of the tasks to be carried out by the person in that position (whether or not employed by the programme). Comparison of the job description with the knowledge and skills of people likely to be available to do a task leads to a list of training needs. A training plan is then prepared from the list of training needs, bearing in mind the priorities of the pro-

**Fig. 10.1. The training cycle**

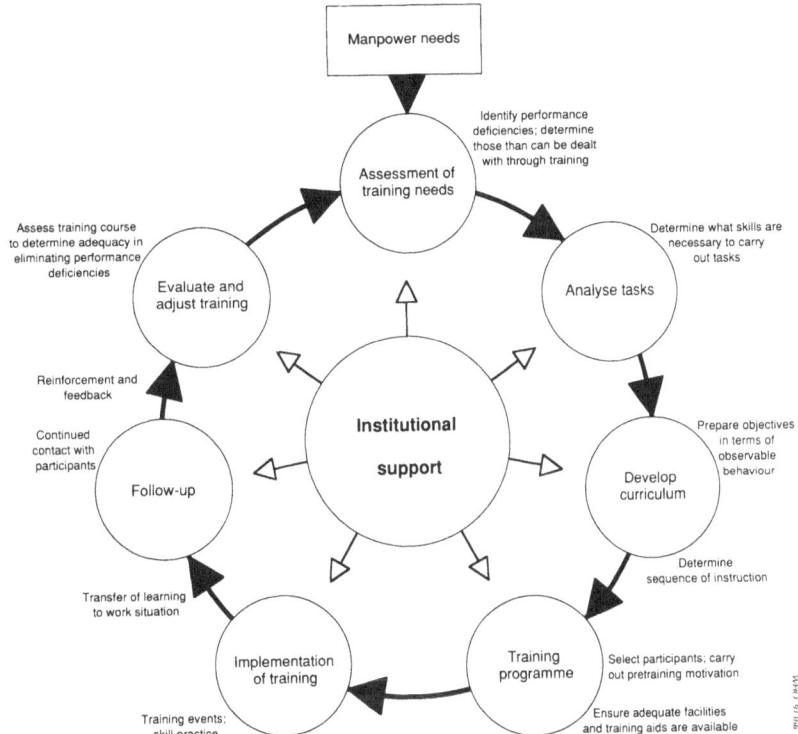

gramme. The plan should specify the people to be trained, with target dates for completion and objectives for what the training should accomplish.

Implementation of training depends on whether the needs are for:

- *knowledge*—where lectures and books are particularly useful;
- *manual skills*—step-by-step development through demonstration, practice and correction of faults, concentrating on key areas;
- *social skills*—use of role-playing, case studies, discussion, practice under supervision;
- *attitude change*—group discussion, personal interview, case studies and feedback; or for
- *systems* (for example clerical procedures and stock control)— check-lists, demonstration and practice with correction.

The final phase of the training cycle is evaluation of what the participants have learned and determination of what they are able to do. This leads to a reassessment of training needs for the next training session or programme. Of course, training and education form a continuous process which starts from what people know and enables them to build upon that foundation of knowledge. There is always opportunity for further learning; it cannot ever be said to have been completed.

## Management requirements

However well people have been trained, they will not be able to reach the objectives of effective sanitation unless their working environment is geared towards meeting those objectives. For example, if there is no transport for project staff to visit sites when required, the community will become disheartened when the expected visitors do not arrive. Similarly, if there is no money to disburse loans to householders when promised, or if there is a lack of supplies, materials and tools, the project will lose momentum. To overcome such problems requires a willingness on the part of management to use all possible means to overcome institutional difficulties.

In addition, project staff, particularly those working directly with the community, require constant encouragement and recognition of their contribution to the project. Suggestions for improving work conditions include:

- regular visits by supervisors and colleagues to those working in isolated situations;
- regular meetings and seminars so that all staff on a project feel part of a team;
- the provision and maintenance of appropriate transport (car, van, motorbike or bicycle);
- alternation of work at rural and urban locations;
- payment of overtime where necessary; and
- ensuring that personnel have occasional postings near their home.

## Motivation

Adequate motivation of agency staff and householders is a prerequisite for successful training. Of particular importance to project staff is the possibility of future career development beyond the present project. If the staff can see a chance of transfer to other projects within a continuous programme, they are more likely to be prepared to learn and improve their skills, and to share their expertise with colleagues and householders. It is important that status, conditions of service and salary scales should compare favourably with those for other available employment. This is particularly important for senior posts where the holders have to work away from home.

# Economic factors

## Choosing between alternatives

Different sanitation techniques may be equally acceptable from the health, social, technical and institutional points of view. The final choice between different techniques is therefore often made on the grounds of cost.

Financial costs, that is, in general terms, what a householder or agency has to pay in cash for a sanitation facility, are discussed on pages 169–176. Economic costs represent the total resource cost to the national economy, that is, what the country as a whole has to pay in terms of labour, materials, health, environment and imports.

Economic comparative costing aims to assign a cost to all the elements that go to make up a system, thus enabling comparisons to be made between competing technologies. It is important for planners and project staff to consider all the alternatives in order to recommend the most economic systems for demonstration and promotion. This then allows the householders to make the final decision on grounds of affordability, convenience and attractiveness.

It should be noted that detailed economic analysis is normally undertaken only for large projects in high-density urban and peri-urban areas. Because of uncertainties in the basic economic data in many countries, it is inadvisable to make final decisions regarding sanitation technology on the basis of economic analysis alone. However, the discipline of thought required to carry out an analysis of the full life-cycle costs of any system can be of great benefit to the planning team by leading to a fuller understanding of all the issues involved.

## Least-cost analysis of alternatives

It is difficult to quantify the benefits obtained from improvements in sanitation. Where there is a choice of technology available to achieve the objective of safe disposal of excreta in an acceptable manner, the benefits obtained from the different options may be presumed to be equivalent. Economic comparison of the alternatives may then be restricted to a "least-cost analysis", which focuses solely on the costs of providing sanitation. There may be variations in the convenience with which this is achieved. For example, a flyless, odourless improved latrine may be far preferable to a flush toilet and septic tank where the water supply is intermittent. However, such situations are so site-specific that it may be generally assumed that the systems outlined in this book (unless specified differently in Chapter 4) have similar benefits with regard to excreta disposal.

Each alternative should be considered according to consistent factors using economic analysis. Non-monetary contributions by householders, for example digging their own pits, should be quantified. Similarly, imported fittings for a pedestal toilet and septic tank should be recorded at their true cost to the national economy, taking into account "real" exchange rates. The values thus assigned may not directly reflect the financial cost involved.

Detailed information on economic analysis and methods of determining "real" values is given in the *Guide to practical project appraisal* (UNIDO, 1978). The main areas that need to be considered are outlined below.

## Economic costs of sanitation systems

### *Labour*

Where a householder is to contribute labour, e.g., by digging the pit or building the superstructure, this work should be costed at the shadow wage rate. This is the rate at which people would be hired to work if there were no artificially controlled wage rates. In a country with high unemployment, the shadow labour rate is likely to be between 40% and 70% of the government minimum wage. Similarly, where agency staff or direct labour is to be used for construction, the costs should be charged at the shadow rate rather than the amount actually to be paid to them. If a labour-only subcontractor is to be employed, the amount to be paid less profit to the subcontractor should be used. Profit represents a "transfer payment" and does not reflect any real transfer of wealth within the economy.

### *Building materials*

The costs of both the superstructure and the substructure must be considered. Where a toilet is to be installed in part of a house, the proportion of the house value represented by the toilet (in terms of the proportion of the floor area) should be included in the calculation.

Building materials may be collected locally without financial charge. There is, however, a labour charge according to the time taken, based on the shadow labour rate. Where the materials to be collected are scarce and efforts are being made to renew them, for example through a reforestation programme, some costs should be assigned to these "free" materials.

For items manufactured in the country, the amount charged by the manufacturer, including transport to the site (less all profit margins), should be used. However, if the item is subsidized by the government, the subsidy should be added to the total cost. Where an item carries a sales tax, the amount of the tax should be subtracted to reflect the real value of the item to the economy.

Where imported items are to be used, the total cost, including freight charges and insurance, should be used, but not including customs duties, local taxes or traders' profits. In some countries, the foreign currency exchange rate may be kept artificially high in order to reduce the financial costs of imports. To reflect the real value of any imported materials, a shadow exchange rate should be used, which is likely to increase the apparent cost of imports. The shadow exchange factor is often in the range 1.2–1.8.

### *Water*

Where water is to be used for flushing the sanitation system, the cost of this water has to be included. If it is to be obtained free of charge from an unimproved source, there is a labour charge for carrying the water to the latrine—calculated from the total time taken, costed at the shadow wage rate. If water is to be obtained from a standpipe or other improved source, the economic cost of delivering that water to the standpipe should be used, in addition to the labour cost of transfer to the latrine. Similarly, where a household has an individual water connection, the economic cost of delivering water to the house must be used. This economic or marginal cost of the extra water used for sanitation is normally higher than the actual tariff paid by the householder. The cost of any pipework and fittings to be used specifically to transfer the water to the toilet should also be considered.

### Land use

Where land is scarce, particularly in urban areas, there is a cost associated with it, which should be included in the analysis.

### Cost of money and the timing of costs

In economic terms, there is a cost involved in using money for one purpose, such as sanitation, as opposed to using it for an alternative purpose. This cost of using money is known as the opportunity cost of capital, and may be defined as the return on an investment in the best alternative use, that is, what could be earned by that money if it was used elsewhere. This cost influences the choice between alternatives with regard to the balance between initial capital investment costs and recurrent operation and maintenance costs. For example, some facilities are expensive to build but cheap to run, while others cost very little to construct but have to be rebuilt and/or emptied at regular intervals.

The influence of the opportunity cost of money on the timing of payments for a sanitation scheme is determined through the mechanism of discounting. This is a technique whereby all future payments made are given a current value by discounting in order to assess fairly the different streams of payments.

In economic analysis, the discount factor is the opportunity cost of capital. Where money invested increases in value over a period of time, the technique of discounting quantifies the money required at the present time in order to obtain a given amount at a set time in the future. Discount factors are normally obtained from tables, but may be calculated directly from the formula:

$$\text{Discount factor} = \frac{1}{(1 + r)^t}$$

where $r$ = discount rate

$t$ = period in years.

The example given on page 173 (example 10.1) demonstrates how the technique might be applied to the practical problems of judging alternative systems.

### Design life of the system

As different facilities are designed to last for different periods, the principles of discounting may also be applied to differing design lives so as to give a fair comparison.

### Emptying and disposal

Pits and tanks may be emptied by hand, for which there are shadow labour charges, or by vacuum tankers, for which there are hourly running costs, including labour, fuel and maintenance. In addition, replacement costs have to be considered, allowing for shadow exchange rates where the machine and spare parts are imported. There is also a cost relating to the disposal of the sludge, whether it is to be discharged to land or to a wastewater treatment plant.

### Groundwater pollution

Wastes that drain through the soil may cause pollution, leading to the need for an alternative water source. If this possibility only applies to one alternative, the possible costs should be estimated and allowed for.

### Sullage disposal

Some systems accept sullage water as well as excreta, thus obviating the need to invest further in sullage removal. This difference should be included where necessary.

### Waste reuse

If the waste products can be reused, for example, sold to farmers as fertilizer or used in a biogas plant, the benefit to be gained should be offset against the costs.

### Governmental and agency management

Most sanitation schemes bear some hidden costs of agency management and promotion. Where alternatives have markedly different charges associated with them, these should be included.

### Analysis

The economic cost of each alternative is determined by calculating all the costs involved in the construction, operation, emptying and maintenance of a particular system over a specified period of time, modified by any appropriate shadow factors. All costs are then discounted by multiplying by a discount factor according to the year in which they will be incurred. This gives the present value of those costs. The present value represents the amount of money required now to be able to pay all expected costs in the future. The present values for each year are then summed to give a single figure of the total present value of the entire life-cycle cash flow, that is, the economic cost for each alternative.

Where alternative systems being compared are expected to last for different periods of time (that is, they have different design lives), it is necessary to take a standard duration in order to make a fair comparison. For on-site sanitation, periods of 10 or 15 years are appropriate. All the costs likely to be incurred during this period for each alternative should be calculated. If the time period is longer than the design life of a system, it is necessary to include rebuilding costs. For a fair comparison it is advisable to choose a standard time that best fits the design life or as nearly as possible a whole multiple of a design life of the alternatives.

Least-cost analysis may be used to compare on-site sanitation with a conventional sewerage system. The nature of the discounting technique, where future costs have a much lower economic impact, tends to favour systems with low initial investment and higher recurrent costs.

## Total annual cost per household

An extension of the least-cost analysis approach is to consider the total annual cost per household (TACH) (Kalbermatten et al., 1982). The initial construction costs are calculated as described above. Because the maintenance costs of most on-site sanitation systems are dependent on the number of people using the system, an average household size appropriate to the area should be selected, usually in the range 6–10 people.

The TACH is calculated by considering the total present value (PV) of the life-cycle cash flow (as described above) as the equivalent of a loan which has to be paid back over the design life of the system at constant, non-inflated prices. The value of yearly repayments, including interest, is obtained by multiplying the present value by a capital recovery factor. This factor is taken from capital recovery factor tables which are based on the equation:

$$\text{Capital recovery factor} = \frac{r(1 + r)^t}{(1 + r)^t - 1}$$

where $r$ = discount rate
$t$ = design life in years

An example of a TACH calculation may be found at the end of this chapter (example 10.2).

Analysis by TACH may be used to compare on-site sanitation systems with conventional sewerage systems. Kalbermatten et al.

167

(1982) calculated that the cost of on-site sanitation was between 5% and 10% of that of conventional waterborne sewerage systems.

## Cost-benefit analysis

Having determined by least-cost analysis the present values of alternative systems, it is normal practice to compare the costs with the present values of the expected benefits. Investment appraisal requires that the present values of benefits should be greater than the present values of the costs. Where alternatives are being considered, the system with the highest margin of benefits over costs should be chosen.

Benefits to be considered include enhanced privacy and convenience for the users, and environmental protection, as well as the reduction and anticipated eventual elimination of excreta-related diseases. Multiple benefits from a single intervention are extremely difficult to isolate and determine, especially where benefits such as improvements in health are interrelated with other basic needs such as nutrition and water supply. Quantification of the benefits of sanitation therefore tends to focus on the more readily measurable reduction of disease and the subsequent increase in productive life expectancy, increase in work capacity, and the reduction of demand for medical facilities and drugs.

Quantification of perceived improvements in the quality of life (for example, not having to squat at the edge of the street before dawn) is based on the value attached to the improvement by the users. Logically this can only be measured by considering the amount people are prepared to pay for those elements of a sanitation system that are most closely related to comfort. However, in most cultures, the investment decisions will be made by men according to their priorities, whereas the greatest benefit is likely to be felt by women who may be unable to declare their preferences.

There are other sanitation benefits to be added, such as reuse of composted or digested excreta for agricultural purposes, or production of biogas for energy needs. However, the benefit to be obtained from this reuse is only occasionally significant.

Quantification of the benefits to be derived from sanitation is extremely difficult. Low-cost sanitation is usually considered as a basic human need, required for human dignity and development as a whole. Economic analysis is therefore best used to compare alternative techniques to determine the least-cost method. This approach is particularly necessary where many of the anticipated environmental or public health benefits will not be realized immediately owing to the necessarily slow pace of community involvement.

A suitable approach to economic analysis is described in the *Guide to practical project appraisal* (UNIDO, 1978) in which it is stated that the literature of project (economic) appraisal commonly gives the impression that the goal is to produce a set of numbers that show whether a project is good or bad but that in reality it is not the numbers themselves that are important, but rather the appreciation of the project's relative strengths and weaknesses that is gained. The numbers are simply an instrument that forces analysts to examine all relevant factors, and a means of communicating their conclusions to others.

## Financial factors

Financial costs represent the money or cash that has to be paid by householders and donor agencies to build and operate a sanitation system (together with allowances for depreciation and bad debts). Financial costs are the main concern of householders and donor agencies whereas economic costs are of greater interest to project planners.

### Financial costs of sanitation systems

#### Labour

Although it is often assumed that the householders can provide much of the labour themselves, this is usually only correct in rural areas. Particularly among disadvantaged groups, such as the disabled, the elderly, and households headed by women in urban areas, skilled and unskilled labour has to be paid for.

#### Building materials

Most items, such as concrete blocks or bricks for pit linings or superstructures, cement for the slabs, water seals, vent pipes, fly screens, roof sheeting and doors, have to be paid for. Only in the rural areas are timber and other materials normally free of cost. Routine maintenance, such as repair of superstructures and renewal of fly screens, will involve costs in the future.

#### Water

For septic tank systems in particular, but also for pour-flush latrines, an allowance must be made for extra payments for the water required for flushing.

#### Cost of money

Interest rates may be payable on loans either at market rates or at subsidized project rates.

#### Emptying and disposal

Allowance should be made for possible future hiring of labourers for the emptying of double pits and the removal of digested sludge, or for the hiring of a vacuum tanker for sludge disposal.

### Waste reuse

In certain limited situations there may be a cash income from selling sludge to farmers.

### Governmental and agency management

Management costs are not normally passed on to householders but remain as a hidden subsidy. Mara (1985b) suggested that the institutional and project delivery costs may be assumed to be about 45% of the sum of labour and material costs.

## Affordability and financial assistance policy

Economic analysis of development projects attempts to show where scarce resources such as capital might be used to best effect. Economic theory requires that, to maximize the benefit to a nation, the financial costs charged to the users should reflect economic costs as closely as possible. However, if the users cannot afford to pay the recommended costs, they will never install a sanitation system and the society as a whole, as well as individual households, will fail to receive the anticipated benefits.

The general policy of international lending agencies is that if the cost of the minimal sanitation facility necessary to ensure adequate health is more than a small part of the household income, then the central or local government should subsidize its construction to make it affordable. Any operation or maintenance costs should be borne by the beneficiary. If, however, some consumers wish to have better or more convenient facilities, they should pay the additional cost themselves. Similarly, if more affluent communities decide that, beyond meeting basic health needs, they wish to safeguard the cleanliness of their rivers or more general environment by building a more expensive sanitation system, they should pay for that system either through direct user charges or through general municipal revenues (Kalbermatten et al., 1982).

Affordability is generally believed to be in the region of 1.5–3% of total household income, that is, total financial costs incurred in a year (initially high investment costs may be spread over a period by use of loans) should not be higher than 3% of total household income for that year. Among the poorest in a poor community, this figure of affordability falls to 1–1.5% of household income.

In many countries, any subsidy of costs over and above this level of affordability has to be rigorously controlled. Development budgets are normally insufficient to subsidize to any significant extent a large number of latrines. There is a danger that small-scale pilot projects with external donor assistance might be given a large subsidy, on the basis of the need to promote the concepts of effective sanitation, when such subsidies could not be extended to a larger scale during expansion of the implementation programme.

There are two other reasons for carefully controlling the level of any subsidy. (1) In some countries, private enterprise can become involved in making and selling the components for sanitation on a large scale. Any subsidy to government projects reduces the profit potential and, therefore, the incentive for private contractors to become involved. Direct subsidies to nongovernment enterprises are usually unacceptable in countries where there is a risk of poor administration. (2) Where a system is not affordable it is usually not maintainable, that is, where the people cannot afford the technology chosen, it is likely that they will also not have the funds to maintain the structure and empty the pits or tanks. The system will then quickly fall into disrepair and the investment will be wasted.

The financial costs of any proposed sanitation system therefore need to be examined very closely. If necessary, installation of pit linings, water seals, vent pipes, cement slabs and superstructures may have to be postponed in order that, at the initial stage, the maximum number of people may benefit from a system which, however simple, leads to a reduction in excreta-related disease.

Where financial subsidies are employed, they should not favour one sanitation system over another in such a way that the economic ranking of alternatives is changed (Kalbermatten et al., 1982).

## Financial assistance

Financial assistance may be necessary to start a sanitation programme and, in countries with appropriate resources, subsidies may be a useful means of quickly propagating public health improvement. Where people cannot afford even the simplest form of sanitation, particularly in urban areas, society as a whole has to pay for the required social benefits through general taxation. However, the use of direct grants is not recommended because of the danger of funds being diverted for purposes other than sanitation.

From India, Roy et al. (1984) suggested that if a programme is designed to serve the poorest groups, a subsidy has to be provided. One method of determining the extent of the subsidy is to use a means test. This may be based on the public utilities (water, electricity, etc.) available in the household. For example, households with no utilities might receive a 75% grant and a 25% loan. Where more utilities are available, the proportion given as a grant decreases. However, even for the poorest households, a small loan component requiring repayment is generally recognized as being vital to ensure effective care and use of the latrines, which only occurs when ownership is clearly vested in the householder rather than the agency.

A revolving fund or loan scheme, whereby money is lent at normal or subsidized interest rates for varying periods of time, may be of great importance. Monthly repayments on loans should be fixed at an affordable level. It is recommended that, if possible, loans for latrines should have a shorter repayment period (for example two years) than loans for housing. This is because benefits perceived by the house-holder are often limited and they may therefore lack motivation to continue payments over a longer period. Where the people have been fully involved in the construction of their latrines, small loans are usually repaid. If a programme is pushed through by an agency without effective community participation, it is likely that there will be a low return.

Revolving funds are a particular form of loan scheme where initial finance from government or a donor is distributed. The fact that there is only a certain amount of money available provides added incentive for borrowers to repay their loans, since other borrowers may have to wait for a loan while their neighbours repay.

There are many possibilities for combining the different types of financial assistance. A government agency might implement and maintain a sanitation system with full or partial cost recovery through tariffs or local taxation. This is more usually the case with a waterborne sewerage system than with on-site sanitation. The householders might do all the work themselves, assisted by grants or loans. They may achieve viable systems simply by accepting advice from external sources. Or the substructure might be constructed by an agency with costs recovered through a tariff, and with the householders building the superstructure with the help of a loan.

Wherever possible, financial assistance should be kept to a minimum, with design and technology appropriate to affordability in the various income groups targeted.

## Costs of sanitation systems

A survey of sanitation by WHO (1987c) suggested that funding limitations are still the most serious constraint on achieving the goal of sanitation for all. The costs of different sanitation systems vary greatly according to country, current exchange rates, and skills needed for designing and implementing on-site technology. The figures given here (from WHO, 1987c, and other sources) are an indication of current costs per person served. However, it should be recognized that these costs are liable to considerable change, even over a short period. The WHO survey discovered increases in median figures between 1980 and 1985 of 131% for individual urban household sanitation in the least developed countries. The survey also noted a 30% decrease in per capita costs for rural sanitation in one region.

In South-East Asia, the per capita cost of sewer connections in urban areas in 1985 varied from US$ 45 to US$ 400 with a median cost of approximately US$ 80. To this must be added an annual water charge in the region of US$ 5 per person served. Low-cost on-site alternatives were costing US$ 13–30 per person in urban areas, and US$ 5–20 per person in rural areas.

In Africa south of the Sahara, sewer connections were reported to cost US$ 120–300 with accompanying water costs in the region of

US$ 8 per year per person. The median sewer connection cost was US$ 150, with urban on-site alternatives ranging from US$ 25 to US$ 70. Rural sanitation costs were in the range US$ 10–45 with a median of US$ 25 per person.

In Central and South America, sewer connection costs varied from US$ 120 to US$ 235 with a median cost of US$ 150, the same as for Africa. Urban on-site sanitation cost US$ 20–80 and rural sanitation ranged from US$ 10 to US$ 50, with an average of about US$ 25 per person served.

## Examples

### Example 10.1. Least-cost analysis

Two alternative on-site sanitation systems (A and B) are to be considered. The discount rate is taken to be 10%, the shadow exchange factor (SEF) for imported goods is 1.3, the shadow wage rate (SWR) for labour is 0.6, and the institutional and promotional costs are 30% of the initial capital cost. All costs are in dollars.

**System A** costs $ 71.80 at the initial construction stage and $ 10 for the use of a vacuum tanker every 5 years. The anticipated life of the system is 20 years. Note: the effects of inflation may be ignored.

| | | Materials | | | Labour | | |
|---|---|---|---|---|---|---|---|
| | | Cost | SEF | Shadow cost | Cost | SWR | Shadow cost |
| Costs of pit: | excavation | | | | 5.00 | 0.6 | 3.00 |
| | lining —bricks | 15.50 | | 15.50 | | | |
| | —cement | 5.00 | 1.3 | 6.50 | | | |
| | construction | | | | 2.00 | 0.6 | 1.20 |
| Costs of slab: | cement | 10.00 | 1.3 | 13.00 | | | |
| | steel reinforcing bar | 3.00 | 1.3 | 3.90 | | | |
| | aggregate | 0.50 | | 0.50 | | | |
| | construction | | | | 2.00 | 0.6 | 1.20 |
| | | 34.00 | | 39.40 | 9.00 | | 5.40 |

| | |
|---|---|
| Total economic cost | 44.80 |
| Cost of superstructure (calculated in a similar manner) | 27.00 |
| Subtotal | 71.80 |
| Cost of institutional support and sanitation promotion (at 30%) | 21.50 |
| Total economic investment cost | 93.30 |

**System B** costs $ 55 for pit, slab and superstructure at the initial stage, with the same amount for a new pit and superstructure after 10 years, at the end of the original design life.

| | |
|---|---|
| Total economic cost | 55.00 |
| Total economic investment cost | 71.50 |
| (calculated in a similar manner to System A above) | |

### Least-cost analysis

| System A | | | | System B | |
|---|---|---|---|---|---|
| Costs (*a*) | Discounted costs (*a*) × DF | Year | Discount factor DF | Costs (*b*) | Discounted costs (*b*) × DF |
| 93.30 | 84.80 | 1 | 0.909 | 71.50 | 65.00 |
| 10.00 | 6.20 | 5 | 0.621 | | |
| 10.00 | 3.90 | 10 | 0.386 | 55.00 | 21.20 |
| 10.00 | 2.40 | 15 | 0.239 | | |
| 123.30 | 97.30 (present value) | | | 126.50 | 86.20 (present value) |

By least-cost analysis, the present value of system B is slightly less than the present value of system A. However, the difference is not enough to allow one system to be chosen in preference to the other on economic grounds alone.

## Example 10.2. Total annual cost per household

The total annual cost per household (TACH) is determined by multiplying the present value of each system by the capital recovery factor (CRF). Using the formula given in the text (page 167), and at an interest rate of 10% over 20 years, CRF = 0.118.

From the figures calculated in Example 10.1:

*System A*
Present value = $ 97.30
TACH = 97.30 × 0.118
= $ 11.50 per household
per year

*System B*
Present value = $ 86.20
TACH = 86.20 × 0.118
= $ 10.20 per household
per year

## Example 10.3. Financial and affordability analysis

Using the figures given in Example 10.1 for system A, it is assumed that the householder is contributing time to excavate the pit and to construct the slab and superstructure.

|  | Financial costs to be paid by household |  |
|---|---|---|
|  | $ |  |
| Labour | 0.00 | (given by household) |
| Bricks | 15.50 |  |
| Cement | 5.00 |  |
|  | 10.00 |  |
| Steel | 3.00 |  |
| Aggregate | 0.00 | (collected by household) |
| Total | 33.50 |  |
| Superstructure | 14.50 | (assumes household labour contribution of 12.50) |
| Total | 48.00 |  |

### Determination of repayments

Assuming a subsidized interest rate of 5% with the loan to be paid off over two years:

Capital recovery factor = 0.538

Annual loan repayments = 0.538 × $ 48.00

= $ 25.80

Check on affordability: annual average household income estimated for this example as $ 380.

$$\text{Repayment as percentage of annual income} = \frac{25.80 \times 100}{380}$$

$$= 6.8\%$$

This would normally be too high for a household to pay, so repayments over four years at a subsidized rate of interest of 3% should be considered:

Capital recovery factor = 0.270

Annual repayments = 0.270 × $ 48.00

= $ 13.00

$$\text{As percentage of annual income} = \frac{13.00 \times 100}{380}$$

$$= 3.4\%$$

This may be acceptable, depending upon the cost of living, and repayments would be completed before the first pit-emptying cost is incurred. As an alternative to subsidizing the rate of interest, it might be possible to sell the latrine slab at a reduced cost. It would be unwise to sell the cement or steel at reduced cost because of the dangers of the materials being used for other purposes. Another alternative is to encourage the use of different building materials to reduce the cost of the superstructure.

Affordability with loan at full rate of interest, repayable over 4 years, slab sold at half price and reduced cost superstructure:

Financial costs
to be paid by household

|  |  | $ |
|---|---|---|
| Labour |  | 0.00 |
| Bricks |  | 15.50 |
| Cement |  | 5.00 |
| Cement }<br>Steel } | as half price slab | 6.50 |
| Aggregate |  | 0.00 |
|  |  | ——— |
| Total |  | 27.00 |
| Superstructure |  | 9.50 (reduced-cost design) |
|  |  | ——— |
| Total |  | 36.50 |

Capital recovery factor $= 0.315$

Annual loan repayments $= 0.315 \times \$ 36.50$

$= \$ 11.50$

Repayment as percentage of annual income $= \dfrac{11.50 \times 100}{380}$

$= 3\%$

## Determination of subsidy

With subsidized rate of interest: assuming a real interest rate of 10%, capital recovery factor $= 0.315$ for four years. Without subsidy, annual repayments would be $ 15.10. With a subsidized rate of interest of 3%, subsidy $= \$ 2.10$ annually for four years in addition to the institutional and promotional costs paid by the agency of approximately $ 22.

With subsidized slab cost: the subsidy represents half the cost of a householder making a slab. Therefore the agency has to pay labour charges as well as half the material costs. Subsidy $= \$ 2.00$, labour and materials $= \$ 6.50$, total subsidy $= \$ 8.50$, in addition to the institutional and promotional costs.

# CHAPTER 11
# Development

Implementation of a successful sanitation project usually follows a recognizable pattern. After the initial surveys, as described in Chapter 9, a demonstration or experimentation phase is required. The demonstration phase is a practical test of the feasibility of the recommended options. This is followed by a consolidation period (Glennie, 1983), primarily to organize the institutional aspects of the project, leading on to the mobilization or expansion phase, when most of the sanitation facilities are constructed.

For the benefit of the agencies involved, it is always advisable to conclude the project with some form of monitoring or evaluation in order to determine how effective it has been. The time scale can vary according to the size of population to be served, its receptivity to development ideas and the financial resources available. However, it is usual to find that the whole sequence takes years rather than months.

## Implementation

The purposes of the preliminary surveys are to determine the extent to which a sanitation programme might be effective and to begin to determine the most appropriate means of meeting public health needs. If the surveys indicate that there is a possibility of a programme being successful, a demonstration phase is required. This phase has three main objectives:

— to identify the techniques and materials that will be most cost-effective;
— to demonstrate the resulting sanitation systems to the community and the government;
— to begin to stimulate demand for sanitation from individual householders.

### Experimental period

An experimental period is normally required for a new sanitation project, during which field staff investigate whether the proposed combination of materials and techniques will work effectively at an affordable level in the particular sociocultural and geographical situation. For example, different systems may need to be compared, and certain elements, such as pit linings, concrete slabs or water seals, may need to be adapted in order to use locally available materials.

Particularly where new techniques or materials are being introduced, the initiators need to carry out a pilot project to work out the technical details to their own satisfaction before promoting the idea to others. Low-income communities cannot afford the risk of installing an unproved system at their own expense.

The period of experimentation also provides an opportunity for informal training of field staff. Those involved in trying out the various alternatives learn the advantages and disadvantages of many different techniques. They can then subsequently explain in convincing detail and from first-hand experience why certain options are being recommended to the prospective users.

If an affordable design is already well recognized and accepted by the prospective users, the experimental phase may be omitted.

### Demonstration

As the project staff gain confidence in the technologies they are promoting, the experimentation period will merge into the demonstration phase, when all interested parties can see the proposed facilities and make their own recommendations and decisions. This enables the promoters to ensure that the technology selected is socially and culturally acceptable to the people. In particular, community representatives and leaders should be given the opportunity to see and discuss the proposals. Results of surveys (which respondents may not always have understood) can be checked against the reality of a demonstration unit.

Government officials from both the sponsoring ministry and related departments and ministries should be encouraged to participate in discussions about the demonstrated systems. Particularly where officials believe that the only acceptable form of sanitation is a high-cost waterborne sewerage system, it is necessary to show that low-cost on-site systems are viable alternatives. Where nongovernmental organizations are involved in the provision of sanitation, it is important that the appropriate government departments have the opportunity to comment at this stage.

The experimental trials are most effective when carried out within the target area at a workshop belonging to the agency or a sympathetic institution, and where prospective users can see the alternatives being tried. The subsequent demonstration sanitation system may be a completed experimental unit or a new system at a new location. The demonstration unit is best installed where local people can try it out in something approaching normal conditions. This may reveal further problems or limitations.

Pilot projects or demonstration systems should be located where people who are committed to the programme can regularly monitor and maintain the latrines. Because a demonstration unit, used by different people, can so easily become fouled, locations that may seem suitable, such as health centres, schools or community buildings, are not always effective sites. More usefully, a health worker's home or the compound of a community development officer who is prepared to care for and maintain the system can be used. Alternatively, the home of a motivated member of the community might be suitable. Where there are village development committees, and particularly where there are water and sanitation committees, prominent members may host demonstration units.

The experimental phase may produce several designs that appear to be suitable for a particular project area. Alternatively, one option that can use a range of different materials may be viable. Variety of design should be encouraged if it enables householders of differing income levels to participate. For example, a ventilated pit latrine can work equally well with a concrete slab or a maintained earth and pole slab. The demonstration phase should show how each solution can be used within the community and at the same time draw attention to possible ways of upgrading the system when financial circumstances permit.

### Stimulating demand

The selection of an appropriate sanitation system should be the responsibility of the people who will ultimately use it. The demonstration phase may be considered as a shop window where potential consumers can see what is on offer at a particular price and determine the model they require. Although most of the selling will go on during the full implementation phase, it is useful, even at this preliminary stage of the project, to begin to stimulate demand.

In many sanitation projects, the public health professionals take a strong lead in initiating the feasibility and demonstration phases. However, the responsibility for successful construction, operation and maintenance should be transferred to the community at the earliest opportunity, preferably before the full implementation or expansion phase starts. Experience has shown that the most successful sanitation projects involve a partnership between the people who will use the scheme and an assisting agency. The agency may be tempted to take too strong a lead role and to attempt to move the programme along too quickly. Working without adequate community involvement may appear to achieve progress in the short term, but it is often to the detriment of the project in the long term.

Wherever possible, low-cost on-site sanitation should be planned and built by the people, operated by the people and maintained by the people. The aim is for minimal agency participation in a community project. As described above, the agency can significantly assist with experimentation and demonstrations to aid people in the decision-making process. The agency can attempt to ensure that the right people have visited demonstration projects. It can help local organizations and government bodies to be aware of the issues by preparing clearly presented documentation. However, to be certain that the people know that the project belongs to them and is under their control, it is important for the agency to restrict its role and not try to direct the project. The community and particularly the individual householders have to sort out their own priorities and move forward at their own pace. This may appear to delay progress and it may frustrate helpers, but true community decisions take time.

Glennie (1983) commented that programmes in which people have been forced to build latrines or where latrines have been provided free of cost have generally failed. "It is essential that a villager builds a latrine only as a result of a conscious decision that he wants to use one. It is the use, rather than the construction, of the latrine that is crucial. The strategy to be adopted therefore, is to encourage at least some villagers to decide that they want to use latrines, thereby stimulating a genuine demand."

In terms of the project cycle, information derived from the demonstration phase concludes the feasibility stage. At this stage, some governments and donor agencies may require an appraisal of the proposals, in the form of an independent check on the work that has been carried out. This appraisal normally covers technical, social, health, environmental, institutional, financial and economic criteria to determine whether the project is well planned and worthy of further investment. On the basis of the appraisal, the donor or government ministry may subsequently approve the decision to proceed with the project. This enables the consolidation phase to commence.

## Consolidation

At the community level the distinction between the demonstration phase and the consolidation phase may appear blurred. However, there comes a point where the basic technology has been proved to be feasible and the project is generally acceptable. Before widespread implementation can begin a period of consolidation is required, primarily to organize the institutional aspects of the project. The demonstration units should continue to be operated and cared for, but the primary thrust at this stage is to determine the support (technical, financial, material and administrative) that the agency will have to provide in order to enable householders to build their own latrines. Training of community personnel and technicians, identification of community leaders, involvement of staff from the health, education and other sectors, confirmation of sanitary codes and regulations, testing of promotional materials, and general administrative support all have to be considered.

### *Governmental approval*

The agency should finalize, as far as possible, the recommended designs for latrines, and seek the widest possible governmental acceptance for the programme. This approval should be sought not only from the institution directly responsible for sanitation but from all interested ministries, councils and committees. However, following on from the demonstration phase and initial contacts with community leaders, the agency and other institutions have to recognize that householders are unlikely to come to a clear-cut decision. Unless the community is unusually homogeneous, it is probable that the people will want a range of options at varying costs. For example, at the simplest level a lined pit could be constructed with a wood and mud slab and only a screen for privacy. At a later date, the household may be able to afford a concrete slab to replace the timber and mud, and then later still a permanent superstructure could be built. On the other hand, some families may be able to afford a concrete slab from the outset.

In certain situations, some latrines may later be upgraded by connection to a main sewerage system, but it is normally impracticable to make specific plans for such improvements in the early stages.

## Institutional support

The flexibility required to meet the differing expectations of house-holders makes the agency's work more difficult. The assistance proffered has to take into account the various income levels and preparedness of the different groups to invest. The agency therefore needs to focus on the aspects of the programme that are crucial to its success. These may be technical, financial, institutional, social or promotional, but the agency would do well not to be diverted into trying to enforce one set solution. In many projects this means that the superstructure, design and construction are left to individual house-holders, while the agency concentrates on general promotional work and helping with slabs and linings along with the water seal (and connecting pipe) or vent pipe, where required.

The approach adopted by the agency must be worked out in advance of widespread promotion within the community so as to minimize any confusion. Whichever approach is taken, standardized procedures should be fixed during the consolidation period. Agency staff can then be trained in these procedures to enable them to give clear and coherent advice to householders.

Any necessary administration required to support the field staff should also be determined on the understanding that it will be there to assist rather than to restrict or limit.

## Training

Sanitarians and technical staff who were not involved in the demon-stration phase should be told about the results and techniques de-veloped earlier. Related staff, such as health workers and sociologists, should also be given an introduction to the programme. The extent of training needed will depend on their proposed role within the pro-gramme, but at the least they should be fully informed as to what is expected of the householders.

Similarly, teachers in local educational establishments should be introduced to the programme and ideally provided with suitable educational material to use with their students. Artisans not directly responsible to the agency but who may become involved as small contractors should be trained in any specialized techniques that may have been developed during the experimentation. Training programmes for householders should be prepared and tested for later use.

### Pre-testing of promotional materials

Any leaflets, plans, posters or other explanatory or promotional material should be pre-tested during the consolidation phase to ensure that the message being received by the readers is the one intended by the promoters. Similarly any teaching materials for schools should also be tested.

### Sanitary codes and regulations

Basic legislation is necessary to enable a public health agency to initiate and develop activities in the field of public health and sanitation. Enabling legislation is normally confined to statements of broad principles, responsibilities and penalties. On the basis of such legislation, the public health agency concerned is in a position to formulate more detailed rules, regulations and standards.

Any existing sanitary code may exert a strong influence on the nature and content of an excreta disposal programme. If the sanitary regulations are outdated, or too elaborate or exacting, they may restrict both the technical and the administrative aspects of the project. Such regulations may defeat their own purpose and are often ignored by the population. When suitably drafted, regulations are useful in helping to ensure a basic minimum of sanitary safeguards and the elimination of potential health hazards, especially in densely populated communities. They usually deal with and prescribe standards for such matters as: the prevention of soil and water pollution; the disposal of human and animal wastes; the hygiene aspects of housing; the protection of food supplies; the control of arthropod, rodent and mollusc hosts of disease; and the use of surface water.

When elaborating sanitary regulations it is important to keep in mind the following principles:

- No regulation should be made that cannot be enforced.
- No law can be enforced without the cooperation of most of the people concerned.

Rules and regulations applying to excreta disposal in low-income areas should be reasonable and no stricter than necessary; above all they should be in accordance with the basic principles of sanitation. It is important to consider every contigency that may occur within the foreseeable future, and the best way to do so is to consult the people for whose benefit the regulations are formulated. While the experience of others may be useful in drafting new regulations, it is always a mistake to adopt the regulations of another country without making necessary modifications.

On the need for the cooperation of the people in the enforcement of legislation, Lethem (1956) wrote, "No form of control can be effective without the support of most of the people concerned, backed by an enlightened public opinion. Hence, education must precede legislation; in fact it might be described as the father of legislation. The lower the standard of education, the greater the need for careful preparation before new regulations can be introduced and enforced. It is better to start in a small way and work up, than to introduce a multiplicity of rules and raise a wall of opposition, which makes enforcement difficult. Legislation alone cannot improve hygiene. To launch regulations without first preparing the way, is like sowing seed without first ploughing the ground. Old traditions die hard, and bad habits are not easy to change."

This statement is particularly applicable to excreta disposal programmes, which are designed to bring about changes in people's attitudes and practices. In this field, public health instruction is more important than compulsion, and sanitary inspection should not have as its primary aim the enforcement of regulations by means of sanctions.

There may be particular areas of concern in existing by-laws which may limit the freedom to introduce low-cost sanitation programmes. For instance, regulations may specify that only water closets connected to a sewer or septic tank are acceptable in urban areas. Other rules may specify a minimum depth for pit latrines which would be unrealistic in particular ground conditions. It is important that these points are amended after full consultation. The most suitable time to make changes is during the consolidation phase, after the various technologies have been tested but before the expansion phase.

Other points to be considered for legislation include the following:

- Defecation in streets and public places should be illegal once sanitary facilities have been made available. Households should be required to install sanitation systems within a specified time of the sanitation programme commencing.
- No new housing developments should be allowed to proceed without suitable sanitation provision.
- The letting of any house or part of a house or household plot for residential purposes without sanitation facilities should be illegal.
- Where a landlord fails to provide sanitation within a specified time, tenants should be empowered to construct facilities and deduct the expense, as agreed with the agency's officers, from the rent payable to the landlord.
- In certain circumstances, local authorities may be empowered to recover loans for construction of latrines from the beneficiaries through local taxation (Roy et al., 1984).

## Mobilization or expansion

The mobilization or expansion phase aims to encourage and enable every householder and institution in the target area to acquire satisfactory sanitation facilities within a certain period of time. This period of expansion may be considered in terms of promotion and construction. Promotion consists of convincing individual householders that they need to improve their sanitation and have the capability to do so. Once the householders make their decision, the individual construction phase begins with particular requirements for support.

### *Promotion*

The mobilization phase is a time of mass communication. It is an opportunity to share information and lessons learnt from the preceding stages with the target group for the programme. Health education to explain the need for sanitation usually has to be stressed as strongly as the proposed solutions. Until people understand the objectives of the project and why sanitation is so important to them, they are unlikely to be fully committed to it. However, in considering the methods of health education and promotion listed below, it is helpful to remember that the primary motivation for sanitation is often the desire for privacy and convenience. Ultimately it has been found that most people choose to improve their sanitation when they see that their neighbour has a clean affordable system which is pleasant to use.

Sanitation may therefore be seen in certain circumstances as a consumer product. The technology that is successful in terms of user take-up has to have some of the attractiveness of any consumer product in addition to being effective and of good value (Franceys, 1987). A valid approach to the promotion of latrines is to consider them as products to be marketed to individual households using all the skills of the advertising and marketing industry.

This approach has been taken in programmes where the experimentation or demonstration workshops have been turned into sanitation centres. These are effectively shops where prospective customers can come to inspect the options available in the various price ranges. They can then discuss with a "salesman" the possibilities of purchasing a system and hear of the special offers open to them regarding technical assistance and financial help. This approach is particularly appropriate for on-site sanitation where each system stands on its own, unconnected to any sewer lines or communal facilities.

A more conventional approach is to consider initial promotion as part of a health education programme which has the following purposes:

● to demonstrate the possibility of improving the health status of the individual and the household;
● to demonstrate the link between well-being, health and sanitation practices;

- to create a desire for improvement in sanitary habits;
- to help determine what changes are needed and desirable for improving sanitation and how they can be implemented;
- to encourage people to put into practice good habits of personal hygiene, and measures to improve personal, home and community sanitary conditions;
- to secure sustained interest and participation in a community programme of environmental health improvement.

There are many methods of promoting health and improved sanitation as a means to health. The ideas listed below should be used in a mixture that suits the culture and aspirations of the people at the time of the programme. It is important to note that the extent of promotional activities should be linked to the agency's capacity to assist with construction of sanitation systems. Otherwise considerable frustration may build up which could be counterproductive.

*Meetings and visits*
Various types of meetings can be used, for example, individual discussions with community leaders, house-to-house visits by community development officers or sanitarians, visits by women health workers to the women in the community, and general public meetings where the wider issues can be discussed by the whole community.

*Role of schools and teachers*
Schoolteachers, especially at primary level, should be trained to prepare the children to use sanitation facilities correctly at school and to understand the need for hygiene and latrines at home. Special lessons should be given to help children understand that a clean water supply with effective sanitation can lead to improved health. This will not only be of benefit to the children but will also serve to reinforce the health message to the community as the children report back to their parents.

*Demonstrations and mass treatment*
Demonstrations may be held using microscopes to show what can be seen in apparently clean water. This is most effective when what is seen can be shown to result from inadequate sanitation. Where such demonstrations can be linked with special clinics to treat people who are ill from excreta-related diseases, a powerful lesson can be provided.

*Community groups*
Selected target groups within the community may be invited to participate in drama or role-playing related to health education and the need for sanitation. Stories and songs can also be effective ways of communicating ideas.

*Leaflets*
Simple technical information leaflets are required, containing illustrations and drawings that have been pre-tested. The leaflets should

describe the different parts of the system, and explain how they work together and how they can be constructed. Written information may also be supplied detailing the help that each household can obtain from the agency. Even if householders are illiterate they are likely to be able to call upon others to explain. It is important that everybody has equal access to details of assistance. Vague promises given at public meetings are not sufficient.

The information given should stress that any solution can eventually be upgraded. Even if householders find that they do not have the required piped water or that they cannot immediately afford the type of sanitation they desire, they should be able to see that there are ways to upgrade their facilities in stages while enjoying the benefits of improved sanitation.

### Training

Ideally, the skills that may be required by local artisans or technicians should be transferred during the consolidation stage. However, where training is also required during the expansion phase, simple practical sessions or demonstrations, where participants construct components and complete systems in selected households in the target area, are effective as a form of promotion as well as training.

### Use of the mass media

There are many forms of the mass media that can be used for promoting specific sanitation options as well as for health education. Their use and the balance between them will depend on the size of the target group, the relative wealth of the people and the availability of funding. Posters, billboards, newspapers, radio, loudspeaker trucks, slides, flip-charts, film, video, and broadcast television have all been used successfully in differing mixes. Careful planning is necessary, as too much information and health education coming too soon may lead to a build-up of resistance against the ideas. Karlin & Isely (1984) considered in detail the use of audiovisual materials for use in sanitation programmes.

Care should be taken to ensure that all the agencies, institutions and health-related bodies have prepared their staff to give the same message. Any conflict between them will lead to mistrust on the part of prospective users.

## Construction

### Selection of system by householders

In the majority of cases individual householders will be responsible for organizing the building of sanitation systems at their own houses. Having chosen the system they feel best fits their needs, they will benefit from continued assistance and support during the construction period.

### Technical assistance

Technical advice regarding the choice of system, the best site for a unit, the depth to which any pit should be dug, and requirements for lining, ventilating, sealing and covering the pit should be available from technicians who can visit the household for detailed discussions. This information should also be available in the form of a written leaflet.

Where required, an auger kit for drilling trial holes may be used by the technical staff to determine the best place to dig the pit.

### Training for householders

Short training sessions may be held at the demonstration workshop to teach householders how to dig and line pits and how to make slabs, vent pipes or seals. Alternatively, householders may be helped to make their own components at the demonstration site.

### Identification of contractors and artisans

Although the skills required for latrine construction are relatively simple, many householders may prefer to pay others to carry out the work. A project can assist by identifying pit excavators, masons or contractors who are trained and able to carry out the work to a satisfactory standard. Agreements and pricing levels may also be negotiated by the agency on behalf of the householders.

### Tools and moulds

Special tools, such as iron bars, pickaxes, spirit levels, or plumb-bobs, that are not normally available in the community, may be provided, for loan, hire or sale. Similarly, reusable moulds for concrete lining rings, slabs or water seals may also be made available by the agency.

### Materials

Where the cost or a shortage of materials necessary for construction causes difficulties, the agency may help with procurement. There is, however, a danger that such materials will be misused, either by incorporation in nonsanitary household building work or through resale to traders. Because of this, materials support is often limited to the provision of precast components of a sanitation system, such as slabs, seals and vent pipes. These may be sold at commercial rates to encourage their production by local businesses, thus fostering industrial development (International Development Research Centre, 1983). Another alternative is to sell at cost price to ensure that people are paying the real cost of their sanitation and to enable a revolving fund to be set up to help others.

Where ventilated pits are recommended, PVC-coated glass fibre or stainless steel fly screens should be readily available from the agency. It is unlikely that householders will be able to purchase such material from local merchants. The alternative mild steel fly screens corrode quickly, giving rise to a significant problem with flies.

### Finance and subsidies

As discussed in Chapter 10, the financial costs to be paid by the householder usually reflect the economic costs (that is, the overall cost to the nation) as closely as possible. However, where it is considered necessary for reasons of social welfare, subsidies may be employed.

Subsidies may be used where the poorest people in the community would not otherwise be able to afford a sanitation system, though care must be taken to ensure this is not simply an excuse to promote inappropriate technology (e.g., to use a more expensive alternative). Subsidies may also be employed where people are unwilling to invest in sanitation because they remain unconvinced as to the benefits to be gained, or where householders are reluctant to invest in what is perceived to be a temporary form of sanitation which does not confer the desired benefits of status and convenience. Finally, subsidies may be used where the agency desires to speed up the development process, to encourage more people to install systems at a faster rate than would otherwise be possible.

The methods used have included subsidized (low-interest) loans for construction of the complete system or loans for the purchase of specific materials or components. These loans usually form part of a revolving fund, set up by a donor, a proportion of which is made available for further projects in other areas. Loans may be totally free of interest or may include a nominal rate of interest to pay overhead charges. Where loans are charged at full commercial rates of interest there is no direct subsidy involved.

A subsidy may also be in the form of a grant for materials or components or as materials or components provided at reduced cost. One approach has been for grants to be made to householders on completion of an acceptable latrine, as an added incentive. Indirect grants may be given in the form of technical assistance or general project assistance which is not charged to the householder. Similarly, some projects may establish shops to sell building materials at cost price, avoiding normal trader profits. There is, however, a subsidy in the form of the overhead costs of the materials store.

The aim of subsidies is to enable householders to construct an acceptable sanitation system at the earliest opportunity. The resultant system has to be at a level where the householder can afford the recurrent costs of operation and maintenance. The level of the subsidy is gauged as the level that enables a sustainable system to be built which is still perceived by the householders as being under their ownership and control.

In India, experience suggests that if a programme is designed to serve the poorest of the poor, a subsidy has to be provided (Roy et al.,

1984). But even for the poorest households, a small loan component requiring repayment is recognized as being vital to ensure effective participation and use of the latrines.

### Site supervision

Information leaflets and training courses alone are not sufficient to ensure that latrines will be built correctly. Technical helpers need to pay visits to households where latrines are being constructed to advise and check on the technical details. Such personnel should provide constructive suggestions and encouragement, rather than negative comments and criticism.

### Institutional support

The lead agency which is promoting sanitation has the major role. However, other government departments, councils, health and educational establishments can also support the project. They should ensure that their own sanitation facilities are adequate for the use of their staff, students and visitors. Such institutions can also assist by providing space for temporary storage of materials.

There are various other forms of institutional support. Government employees have been given time off from work to construct their own sanitation systems as a model for their neighbours to copy. Similarly, it has been known for a government to declare a public holiday for all employees, both private and public, to spend time building latrines. However, there is a strong likelihood that the results of such special events will be less than hoped for unless the correct preparation (surveys and demonstrations) has been done.

### Loan repayments

Monthly instalments to pay back loans should be fixed at levels that are affordable rather than at rates designed to ensure quick repayment. However, this has to be balanced by the need to ensure that repayment periods are not excessive, since householders may be reluctant to continue paying over a long period for a facility such as sanitation.

Where the people have been fully involved in the construction of their latrines, it is usual to find that small loans for latrine construction are repaid. If a programme is forced through by an agency without full community involvement, it is likely that there will be a low return rate on loans.

### Completion of the programme

Within most programmes, the rate of completion of individual sanitation units tends to follow an "S" curve (Fig. 11.1). In the initial demonstration and consolidation phases there is little progress in terms

**Fig. 11.1. Pattern of installation of latrines in a sanitation programme**

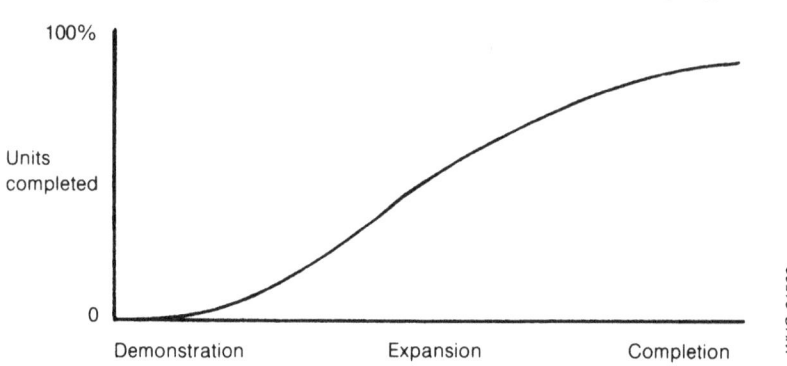

of numbers of systems completed. During the expansion phase the majority of the population are expected to install latrines. However, the rate of installation normally falls as the 80% completion level is neared. During the completion stage additional positive inducements should not be used, since this would be unfair to those who have already constructed their facilities on their own. Unless the failure to complete is due to particular social disadvantage, in urban and periurban areas legal action may have to be taken to ensure completion by all households. As the health benefits cannot be fully realized unless all members of the community use improved sanitation (particularly in areas of high population density), it is reasonable to expect substantial compliance.

There are many different approaches to assisting householders to construct their own sanitation facilities. For each project the right mix of assistance, motivation and legislation has to be determined in order to produce the desired results.

## Operation and maintenance

### Household responsibility

Completion of latrine construction marks the beginning of the real sanitation programme in that it is the point at which people can start to realize the benefits of their investment. Continuing health education and technical assistance are required to ensure that new systems function properly. For example, longer-term assistance may be required to ensure that double pits are emptied and used in rotation.

Some householders may benefit from advice as to how to encourage all members of their family to use the facility in a clean and safe way. Laver (1986) described how local potters were taught to make ceramic tiles depicting good habits of latrine use, which could be fixed permanently on the latrine walls to act as a constant reminder of good practice.

Use of hard cleaning materials such as stones and corncobs leads to increased rate of sludge accumulation, and hence to a shortened life for the pit or tank before emptying or to blockages in water seals or pipes.

Members of the community should be told about the effects of using such bulky cleansing materials, and encouraged to find alternatives. Where it is not the custom to use water for anal cleansing, leaves, grass or paper are preferable. Details of the maintenance required for different types of latrine can be found in Chapter 6.

The latrine superstructure, like all buildings, needs regular maintenance to ensure that it remains structurally sound and pleasing to use.

Responsibility for maintenance must never be left undecided until the need becomes apparent. By that time many people will have stopped using the facility and returned to their old places. The latrine itself may have become so unpleasant that it is more difficult to find somebody to care for it regularly. Maintenance becomes a particular problem where an agency has been constructing sanitation systems for people without their full involvement in planning and design. If householders are unsure of the ownership of the system they are less likely to accept responsibility for looking after it.

## Agency responsibility

The householder or user has primary responsibility for using and maintaining the latrine. The agency may have to assist in two areas: (1) ensuring the availability of special items such as vent-pipe screening; and (2) the provision of services requiring special equipment, such as pit emptying. Initial demand may not be sufficient for private traders to stock specialized vent screening or plastic water seals. While this demand builds up, the agency should ensure that such items may still be purchased from a public health department after completion of the construction phase. Where double pits are used, the householder should empty the pit at regular intervals, using the dry sludge on the land as a fertilizer. Where single pits require mechanical emptying, particularly in urban areas, an organization should be established or the local council should run vacuum tankers at an affordable cost to the householder.

## Evaluation

As a sanitation project nears the end of the implementation phase, it is helpful to carry out an evaluation or review of what has occurred. Evaluation, by personnel who have not been directly involved with the project, is only of relevance to the community if the agency is prepared to correct any mistakes identified, particularly those of a technical nature that may lead to difficulties with operation or maintenance in later years. Evaluation is important for the agency, as it gives staff a better understanding of what has been effective and why, and at the same time pinpoints any failures that could be avoided in future programmes.

In the sense that evaluation is an ongoing management tool to ensure effective use of resources, it is sometimes considered necessary to engage in constant evaluation of all stages of a programme. Regular monitoring should be carried out as routine by the management of any agency involved. Constant evaluation is normally only justified in large programmes. Evaluation carried out during or at the end of the project should be done by people who are familiar with the project or other similar projects but who have not been closely associated with the planning and implementation. This is to avoid the natural tendency for people to make allowances for shortcomings and weaknesses in any scheme with which they have been involved.

Because of the pressures on project budgets and professional staff time, the evaluation has to give the required information at minimum cost. Occasionally it may be of interest to carry out a number of evaluations over a period of years subsequent to completion of the project. However, the results rarely justify the costs involved.

The World Health Organization has developed a minimum evaluation procedure (MEP) for water supply and sanitation projects (WHO, 1983). In this, evaluation is defined as "a systematic way of learning from experience and of using the lessons learned both to improve the planning of future projects and also to take corrective action to improve the functioning, utilization and impact of existing projects." Using the MEP, the first consideration is how effectively the facilities are working or functioning. This is followed by an investigation as to how well the sanitation system is being used and maintained by the people; and finally the impact on the health and welfare of the community is considered. A protocol for inspection of latrines, included in the MEP, is shown in Fig. 11.2.

Evaluation normally leads to recommendations for further action to improve the effectiveness of sanitary facilities. There should be a readiness within the programme institutions to make the recommended alterations if the time and expense of carrying out the evaluation are to be justified.


## Functioning

Evaluation of functioning, that is, determination of how well the different systems are working, can be considered in terms of the proportion of households in the target area who have constructed a sanitation system, and the reliability of the facilities (Fig. 11.3). Failure to reach at least 80% of the target population may be because the facilities are unaffordable or are not considered of immediate priority by the community in terms of expected benefits.

Technical confusion over the design, use of inappropriate materials, a high groundwater table and hard rock all lead to a lower than anticipated response. Where the facilities are unhygienic (for example, because of constant fouling, flooding or fly nuisance), reasons for this failure should be investigated. Reliability should be considered in terms of operation and maintenance, rate of filling of pits, convenience of

**Fig. 11.2. Protocol for the inspection of latrines**

Programme: _____    Province: _____
                                         District: _____
                                         Village: _____
                                         Inspected by: _____
                                         Date: _____

1. Household identification            _____

2. Superstructure, type                _____

                                       Yes        No
   Functioning                         _____  _____
   Gives privacy                       _____  _____
   Gives protection from rain          _____  _____

3. Fixtures, type                      _____

                                       Yes        No
   Water in water seal                 _____  _____
   Lid                                 _____  _____
   Suitable                            _____  _____
   If not suitable specify problem     _____

                                       Yes        No
4. Pit lined                           _____  _____
   Free depth _____ metres

                                       Yes        No
5. Cleaning material available         _____  _____

6. Water for handwashing available at what distance? _____ metres

7. General condition

                        Good    Acceptable    Bad    Very bad
   Smell                _____  _____   _____  _____
   Flies                _____  _____   _____  _____
   Mosquitos            _____  _____   _____  _____
   Fouling              _____  _____   _____  _____

8. Other comments

   _____

   _____

   _____

*WHO 91501*

superstructures, and functioning of items such as water seals and vent pipes.

## Utilization

In recording the proportion of people using the systems, particular attention should be paid to the different categories in the community, such as women, men, children and old people. However, such information is often difficult to collect, as people may give replies they think the

**Fig. 11.3. Evaluation of sanitation facilities**

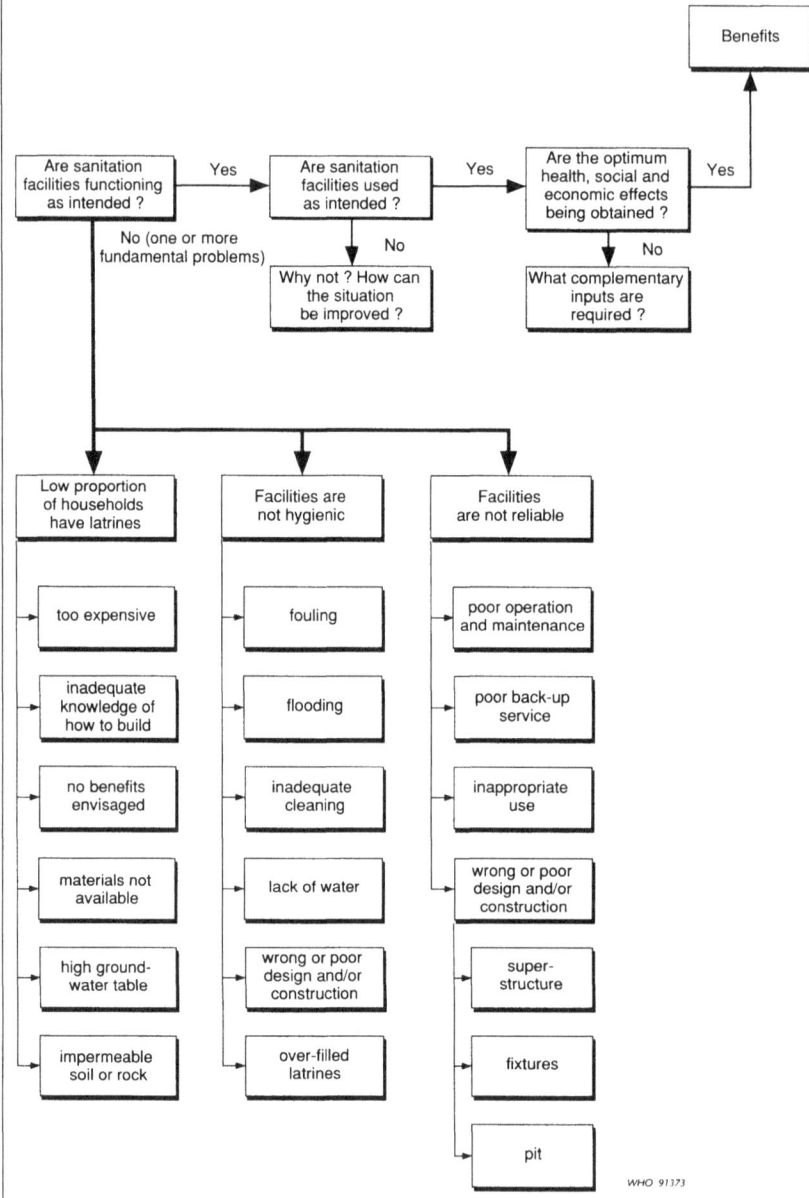

WHO 91373

evaluator requires. Watching who uses a latrine may be considered an invasion of privacy. A careful combination of interviewing and observation is needed. Low rates of use may be due to technical inadequacies, sociological issues, lack of health education, or a general uncertainty regarding the system. It is important to distinguish between these different factors.

## Health impact

Evaluation of health impact is only worth while when the factors hindering functioning and utilization have been overcome. The aim is to determine whether there has been any improvement in health and well-being as a result of the sanitation programme. Such studies tend to be expensive and normally require specially trained personnel such as medical officers and epidemiologists. Briscoe et al. (1986) gave detailed information on the complexities of measuring health impact. In particular, the authors looked at the conditions under which health impact evaluations should be carried out, the preferred indicators for measuring impact on health, appropriate methods for study, and means of interpreting the results. They concluded that such detailed evaluations are justified where further large investments are contemplated and economic criteria are not sufficient to decide between alternative options, where systems are functioning and being utilized, and where sufficient resources (including scientific personnel) are available.

The ultimate evaluation is that of the householders themselves. A project can be considered successful where householders, by their own choice, have invested a significant amount of time and money in the implementation of their own sanitation systems, and demonstrate their satisfaction by their continued willingness to use, operate and maintain their latrines.

# References

ALUKO, T. M. (1977) Soil percolation tests in the Lagos area. *Journal of the Institution of Public Health Engineers*, 5 (6): 152–155.

ASSOCIAÇÃO BRASILEIRA DE NORMAS TÉCNICAS (1982) *Construcao e instalcao de fossas septicas e disposicao dos efluentes finais*. Rio de Janeiro (NBR 7229).

BALASEGARAM, M. & BURKITT, D. P. (1976) Stool characteristics and western diseases. *Lancet*, 1: 152.

BASKARAN, T. R. (1962) *A decade of research in environmental sanitation*. New Delhi, Indian Council on Medical Research (Special Report Series No. 40).

BERG, A. (1973) *The nutrition factor and its role in national development*. Washington, DC, Brookings Institution.

BLUM, D. & FEACHEM, R. G. (1983) Measuring the impact of water supply and sanitation investments on diarrhoeal diseases: problems of methodology. *International journal of epidemiology*, 12 (3): 357–365.

BOESCH, A. & SCHERTENLEIB, R. (1985) *Emptying on-site excreta disposal systems: field tests with mechanized equipment in Gaborone (Botswana)*. Dübendorf, Switzerland, International Reference Centre for Waste Disposal (IRCWD Report No. 03/85).

BRADLEY, R. M. (1983) The choice between septic tanks and sewers in tropical developing countries. *The public health engineer*, 11 (1): 20–28.

BRANDBERG, B. (1985) Why should a latrine look like a house? *Waterlines*, 3: 24–26.

BRISCOE, J. (1984) Water supply and health in developing countries: selected primary health care revisited. *American journal of public health*, 74 (9): 1009–1013.

BRISCOE, J. ET AL. (1986) *Evaluating health impact: water supply, sanitation, and hygiene education*. Ottawa, International Development Research Centre.

BRITISH STANDARDS INSTITUTION (1972) *Code of practice: small sewage treatment works*. London (CP302).

VAN BURNE, A. ET AL. (1984) Composting latrines in Guatemala. *Ambio*, **13** (4): 274–277.

BURKITT, D. P. ET AL. (1974) Dietary fibre and diseases. *Journal of the American Medical Association*, **229**:1068–1074.

BUTLER, R. G. ET AL. (1954) Underground movement of bacterial and chemical pollutants. *Journal of the American Water Works Association*, **46** (2):97–111.

CAIRNCROSS, S. & FEACHEM, R. G. (1983) *Environmental health engineering in the tropics: an introductory text*. Chichester, Wiley.

CALDWELL, E. L. (1937) Pollution flow from pit latrines when impervious stratum closely underlines the flow. *Journal of infectious diseases*, **61**:270–288.

CAREFOOT, N. F. (1987) Human resources development. In: *Developing world water*, Vol. 2. London, Grosvenor Press International.

CARROLL, R. F. (1985) Mechanised emptying of pit latrines in Africa. In: Ince, M., ed., *Proceedings of the eleventh WEDC Conference: Water and sanitation in Africa*. Loughborough, Water, Engineering and Development Centre, pp. 29–32.

CHEESBROUGH, M. (1984) *Medical laboratory manual for tropical countries. Volume II: Microbiology*. Sevenoaks, Kent, Tropical Health Technology.

COTTERAL, J. A. & NORRIS, D. P. (1969) Septic tank systems. *Journal of the environmental engineering division, Proceedings of the American Society of Civil Engineers*, **95**:715–746.

CRANSTON, D. & BURKITT, D. P. (1975) Diet, bowel behaviour and disease. *Lancet*, **2**:37.

CROFTS, T. J. (1975) Bowel-transit times and diet. *Lancet*, **1**:801.

CURTIS, C. F. & HAWKINS, P. M. (1982) Entomological studies of on-site sanitation systems in Botswana and Tanzania. *Transactions of the Royal Society of Tropical Medicine and Hygiene*, **78** (1):99–108.

DENYER, S. (1978) *African traditional architecture*. London, Heinemann.

EGBUNWE, N. (1980) Alternative excreta disposal systems in Eastern Nigeria. In: Pickford, J. & Ball, S., ed. *Water and waste engineering in Africa. Proceedings of the sixth WEDC Conference*. Loughborough, Water, Engineering and Development Centre, pp. 137–140.

FEACHEM, R. G. ET AL. (1983) *Sanitation and disease: health aspects of excreta and wastewater management*. Chichester, Wiley.

5555

5

FRANCEYS, R. (1987) Sanitation for low income housing, Juba, Sudan. In: *African Water Technology Conference, Nairobi*. London, World Water, pp. 141–149.

GEYER, J. C. ET AL. (1968) *Water and wastewater engineering*, Vol. 2. New York, Wiley.

GLENNIE, C. (1983) *Village water supply in the Decade: lessons from field experience*. Chichester, Wiley.

GROVER, B. (1983) *Water supply and sanitation project preparation handbook: Vol. 1: Guidelines*. Washington, DC, World Bank (World Bank Technical Paper No. 12).

HUTTON, L. G. ET AL. (1976) A report on nitrate contamination of groundwaters in some populated areas of Botswana. Lobatse, Botswana, Geological survey (unpublished report BGSD/8/76).

INTERNATIONAL DEVELOPMENT RESEARCH CENTRE (1983) *The latrine project, Mozambique*. Ottawa (IDRC-MR58e).

JEEYASEELAN, S. ET AL. (1987) *Low-cost rural sanitation—problems and solutions*. Bangkok, Environmental Sanitation Information Center.

KALBERMATTEN, J. M. ET AL. (1980) *Appropriate technology for water supply and sanitation: a planner's guide*. Washington, DC, World Bank.

KALBERMATTEN, J. M. ET AL. (1982) *Appropriate sanitation alternatives: a technical and economic appraisal*. Baltimore, Johns Hopkins University Press.

KARLIN, B. & ISELEY, R. B. (1984) *Developing and using audio-visual materials in water supply and sanitation programs*. Arlington, Water and Sanitation for Health Project (WASH Technical Paper No. 30).

KHANNA, P. N. (1985) *Indian practical civil engineer's handbook*. New Delhi, Engineers' Publishers.

KIBBEY, H. J. ET AL. (1978) Use of faecal streptococci as indicators of pollution of soil. *Applied and environmental microbiology*, 35 (4):711–717.

LAAK, R. (1980) Multichamber septic tanks. *Journal of the environmental engineering division, Proceedings of the American Society of Civil Engineers*, 106:539–546.

LAAK, R. ET AL. (1974) Rational basis for septic tank system design. *Ground water*, 12:348–352.

LAVER, S. (1986) Communications for low-cost sanitation in Zimbabwe. *Waterlines*, 4 (4):26–27.

LETHEM, W. A. (1956) *The principles of milk legislation and control.* Rome, Food and Agriculture Organization of the United Nations (Agricultural Development Paper, No. 59).

LEWIS, W. J. ET AL. (1980) The pollution hazard to village water supplies in eastern Botswana. *Proceedings of the Institution of Civil Engineers,* **69**: 281–293.

McCARTY, P. (1964) Anaerobic waste treatment fundamentals, part 1. *Public works,* **95**: 107–112.

McCLELLAND, I. & WARD, J. S. (1976) Ergonomics in relation to sanitaryware design. *Ergonomics,* **19** (4): 465–478.

MacDONALD, O. J. S. (1952) *Small sewage disposal systems.* London, Harrison & Crosfield.

McMICHAEL, J. K. (1976) *Health in the third world . . . studies from Vietnam.* London, Spokesman Books.

MAJUMDER, N. ET AL. (1969) A critical study of septic tank performance in rural areas. *Journal of the Institute of Engineers (India),* **40** (12): 743–761.

MARA, D. D. (1984) *The design of ventilated improved pit latrines.* Washington, DC, World Bank (TAG Technical Note No. 13).

MARA, D. D. (1985a) *Ventilated improved pit latrines: guidelines for the selection of design options.* Washington, DC, World Bank (TAG Discussion Paper No. 4).

MARA, D. D. (1985b) *The design of pour-flush latrines.* Washington, DC, World Bank (TAG Technical Note No. 15).

MARA, D. D. & CAIRNCROSS, S. (1989) *Guidelines for the safe use of wastewater and excreta in agriculture and aquaculture.* Geneva, World Health Organization.

MARA, D. D. & SINNATAMBY, G. S. (1986) Rational design of septic tanks in warm climates. *The public health engineer,* **14** (4): 49–55.

MORGAN, P. R. (1977) The pit latrine—revived. *Central African journal of medicine,* **23**: 1–4.

MORGAN, P. R. & MARA, D. D. (1982) *Ventilated improved pit latrines: recent developments in Zimbabwe.* Washington, DC, World Bank (World Bank Technical Paper No. 3).

NITRATE COORDINATION GROUP (1986) *Nitrates in water.* London, HMSO (Pollution Paper No. 26).

OLDCORN, R. (1982) *Management—a fresh approach.* London, Pan Books.

PACEY, A., ed. (1978) *Sanitation in developing countries.* Chichester, Wiley.

PACEY, A. (1980) *Rural sanitation: planning and appraisal.* London, IT Publications.

PARRY, J. (1985) *Fibre concrete roofing.* West Midlands, Intermediate Technology Workshops.

PHADKE, N. S. ET AL. (undated) *Study of a septic tank at Borivli, Bombay.* Bombay, CPHERI Bombay Zonal Laboratory.

PICKFORD, J. (1980) *The design of septic tanks and aqua-privies.* Garston, Building Research Establishment (Overseas Building Note No. 187).

PRADT, L. A. (1971) Some recent developments in night-soil treatment. *Water research,* 5: 507–521.

REYNOLDS, C. E. & STEEDMAN, J. C. (1974) *Reinforced concrete designers' handbook.* London, Viewpoint.

ROY, A. K. ET AL. (1984) *Manual on the design, construction and maintenance of low-cost pour-flush waterseal latrines in India.* Washington, DC, World Bank (TAG Technical Note No. 10).

RYAN, B. A. & MARA, D. D. (1983) *Ventilated improved pit latrines: vent pipe design guidelines.* Washington, DC, World Bank (TAG Technical Note No. 6).

RYBCZYNSKI, W. (1981) *Double vault composting toilets: a state of the art review.* Bangkok, Environmental Sanitation Information Center (ENSIC Review No. 6).

SANCHES, W. R. & WAGNER, E. G. (1954) Experience with excreta disposal programmes in rural areas of Brazil. *Bulletin of the World Health Organization,* 10: 229–249.

SCOTT, J. C. (1952) *Health and agriculture in China: a fundamental approach to some of the problems of world hunger.* London, Faber & Faber.

SHAW, V. A. (1962) A system for the treatment of nightsoil and conserving tank effluent in stabilization ponds. In: *Proceedings of the twentieth Annual Health Congress.* East London, South Africa, Institute of Public Health.

SIMPSON-HEBERT, M. (1984) Water and sanitation: cultural considerations. In: Bourne, P. G., ed., *Water and sanitation: economic and sociological perspectives.* Orlando, Academic Press.

SRIDHAR, M. K. C. ET AL. (1981) Health hazards and pollution from open drains in a Nigerian city. *Ambio,* 10: 29–33.

STUMM, W. & MORGAN, J. J. (1981) *Aquatic chemistry.* New York, John Wiley & Sons.

TACK, C. H. (1979) *Preservation of timber for tropical building*. Garston, Building Research Establishment (Overseas Building Note No. 183).

TANDON, R. K. & TANDON, B. N. (1975) Stool weight in northern Indians. *Lancet*, 2:560–561.

TRUESDALE, G. A. & MANN, H. (1968) Synthetic detergents and septic tanks. *Surveyor and municipal engineer*, 131:28–33.

UNCHS (undated) *Building with bamboo*. Nairobi, United Nations Centre for Human Settlements (UNCHS Technical Note No. 4).

UNITED NATIONS CHILDREN'S FUND (1986) *The state of the world's children 1986*. New York.

UNITED NATIONS DEVELOPMENT PROGRAMME (undated) *Decade dossier*. New York, UNDP Division of Information.

UNIDO (1978) *Guide to practical project appraisal*. New York, United Nations.

US DEPARTMENT OF HEALTH, EDUCATION, AND WELFARE (1969) *Manual of septic tank practice*. Washington, DC (PHS No. 526).

US ENVIRONMENTAL PROTECTION AGENCY (1980) *Design manual: on site wastewater treatment and disposal systems*. Cincinnati, OH, Office of Research and Development, Municipal Environmental Research Laboratory.

WAGNER, E. G. & LANOIX, J. N. (1958) *Excreta disposal in rural areas and small communities*. Geneva, World Health Organization (WHO Monograph Series No. 39).

WAGNER, E. G. & LANOIX, J. N. (1959) *Water supply for rural areas and small communities*. Geneva, World Health Organization (WHO Monograph Series No. 42).

WALSH, J. A. & WARREN, K. S. (1979) Selective primary health care. *New England journal of medicine*, 301:967–974.

WEIBEL, S. R. ET AL. (1949) *Studies on household sewage disposal systems; Part 1*. Cincinnati, OH, Environmental Health Center.

WILSON, J. G. (1987) The development of an appropriate vacuum tanker. In: *African Water Technology Conference, Nairobi*. London, World Water.

WINBLAD, U. & KALAMA, W. (1985) *Sanitation without water*. Basingstoke, Macmillan.

WHO (1950) *Expert Committee on Environmental Sanitation*: report on the first session. Geneva, World Health Organization (WHO Technical Report Series, No. 10).

WHO (1954) *Expert Committee on Environmental Sanitation*: third report. Geneva, World Health Organization (WHO Technical Report Series, No. 77).

WHO (1983) *Minimum evaluation procedure (MEP) for water supply and sanitation projects.* Unpublished document ETS/83.1.[a]

WHO (1984) *Guidelines for drinking water quality*, Vol. 1–3. Geneva, World Health Organization.

WHO (1985) *The control of schistosomiasis*: report of a WHO Expert Committee. Geneva, World Health Organization (WHO Technical Report Series, No. 728).

WHO (1986) *The International Drinking Water Supply and Sanitation Decade Directory: Review of National Progress (as at December 1983)* (WHO CWS Series of Cooperative Action for the Decade).[a]

WHO (1987a) *Technology for water supply and sanitation in developing countries*: report of a WHO Study Group. Geneva, World Health Organization (WHO Technical Report Series, No. 742).

WHO (1987b) *Prevention and control of intestinal parasitic infections*: report of a WHO Expert Committee. Geneva, World Health Organization (WHO Technical Report Series, No. 749).

WHO (1987c) *Review of mid-Decade progress (December 1985)*. Unpublished document CWS/87.5.[a]

WHO (1989) *Health guidelines for the use of wastewater in agriculture and aquaculture*: report of a WHO Scientific Group (WHO Technical Report Series, No. 778).

WHO (1990) *The International Drinking Water Supply and Sanitation Decade. Review of decade progress (as at December 1988)*. Unpublished document WHO/EHE/CWS/90.16.[a]

YEAGER, J. G. & O'BRIEN, R. I. (1979) Enterovirus inactivation in soil. *Applied and environmental microbiology*, 38:694–701.

DE ZOYSA, I. ET AL. (1984) Perceptions of childhood diarrhoea and its treatment in rural Zimbabwe. *Social science and medicine*, 19:727–734.

[a] Available on request from Division of Environmental Health, World Health Organization, 1211 Geneva 27, Switzerland.

# Selected further reading

ASHWORTH, J. (1982) Urban sullage in developing countries. *Waterlines*, 1 (2):14–16.

BOURNE, P. G., ed. (1984) *Water and sanitation: economic and sociological perspectives*. Orlando, Academic Press.

CROSS, P. (1985) Existing practices and beliefs in the use of human excreta. *IRCWD news*, 23:2–4.

DECK, F. L. O. (1986) Community water supply and sanitation in developing countries, 1970–1990: an evaluation of the levels and trends of services. *World health statistics quarterly*, 39 (1):2–39.

EDWARDS, P. (1985) *Aquaculture: a component of low cost sanitation technology*. Washington, DC, World Bank (World Bank Technical Paper No. 36).

ELMENDORF, M. & BUCKLES, P. (1980) *Socio-cultural aspects of water supply and excreta disposal*. Washington, DC, World Bank.

GOLLADAY, F. L. (1983) *Appropriate technology for water supply and sanitation: meeting the needs of the poor for water supply and sanitation*. Washington, DC, World Bank.

GOTAAS, H. B. (1956) *Composting: sanitary disposal and reclamation of organic wastes*. Geneva, World Health Organization (WHO Monograph Series No. 31).

GUNNERSON, C. G. & STUCKEY, D. C. (1986) *Anaerobic digestion: principles and practice of biogas systems*. Washington, DC, World Bank (World Bank Technical Paper No. 49).

HEALEY, K. A. & LAAK, R. (1974) Site evaluation and design of seepage fields. *Journal of the environmental engineering division, Proceedings of the American Society of Civil Engineers*, 100:1133–1146.

HINDHAUGH, G. M. A. (1973) Night soil treatment. *Consulting engineer*, 37 (9):47, 49.

INTERNATIONAL DEVELOPMENT RESEARCH CENTRE (1981) *Sanitation in developing countries. Proceedings of a workshop on training held in Lobatse, Botswana, 14–20 August 1980*. Ottawa (IDRC-168e).

INDIAN STANDARDS INSTITUTION (1969) *Code of practice for design construction of septic tanks*. New Delhi (IS 2470, part 1 and part 2)

LECLERE, M. & SHERER, K. (1984) *A workshop design for latrine construction: a training guide.* Arlington, Water and Sanitation for Health Project (WASH Technical Report No. 25).

LEWIS, W. J. ET AL. (1982) *The risk of groundwater pollution by on-site sanitation in developing countries: a literature review.* Dübendorf, Switzerland, International Reference Centre for Waste Disposal (IRCWD Report No. 01/82).

MCGAUHEY, P. H. & KRONE, R. B. (1967) *Soil mantle as a wastewater treatment system.* Sanitary Engineering Research Laboratory, University of California.

NICOLL, E. H. (1974) Aspects of small water pollution control works. *Journal of the Institute of Public Health Engineers*, **12**:185–211.

VAN NOSTRAND, J. & WILSON, J. G. (1983a) *The ventilated improved double-pit latrine: a construction manual for Botswana.* Washington, DC, World Bank (TAG Technical Note No. 3).

VAN NOSTRAND, J. & WILSON, J. G. (1983b) *Rural ventilated improved pit latrines: a field manual for Botswana.* Washington, DC, World Bank (TAG Technical Note No. 8).

PARLATO, R. (1984) *A monitoring and evaluation manual for low-cost sanitation programs in India.* Washington, DC, World Bank (TAG Technical Note No. 12).

PATHAK, B. (1981) *Sulabh Shauchalaya (hand flush water seal latrine): a simple idea that worked.* Patna, India, Amolla Prakashan.

PEEL, C. (1977) The public health and economic aspects of composting night soil with municipal refuse in tropical Africa. In: Pickford, J., ed., *Planning for water and waste in hot countries. Proceedings of the third WEDC Conference.* Loughborough, Water, Engineering and Development Centre, pp. 25–36.

RAMAN, V. ET AL. (1969) Secondary treatment and disposal of effluent from septic tanks. 4. Preliminary studies of treatment by upward (reverse flow) rock filters. *Journal of the Institute of Engineers (India)*, **49** (6):90–93.

SAGAR, G. & JAIN, A. K. (1982) Ferrocement septic tanks. *Journal of ferrocement*, **12** (1):63–69.

SANDERS, A. & CARVER, R. (1985) *The struggle for health.* Basingstoke, Macmillan.

SHUVAL, H. I. ET AL. (1981) *Night-soil composting.* Washington, DC, World Bank (Appropriate technology for water supply and sanitation, Vol. 10).

US PUBLIC HEALTH SERVICE (1933) The sanitary privy. Washington, DC (revised type No. IV of *Public health report* (Wash), Suppl. 108).

VINCENT, L. J. ET AL. (1961) A system of sanitation for low cost high density housing. In: *Proceedings of a symposium on hygiene and sanitation in relation to housing, Niamey*, pp. 135–172 (Publication No. 84, CETA/WHO, Niger).

WHO (1980) *Epidemiology and control of schistosomiasis*: report of a WHO Expert Committee. Geneva, World Health Organization (WHO Technical Report Series, No. 643).

WHO REGIONAL OFFICE FOR SOUTH-EAST ASIA (1985) *Achieving success in community water supply and sanitation projects*. New Delhi (Regional Health Paper No. 9).

VAN WIJK-SIJBESMAN, C. (1985) *Participation of women in water supply and sanitation: roles and realities*. The Hague, International Reference Centre for Community Water Supply and Sanitation (IRC Technical Paper No. 22).

# Glossary of terms used in this book

**adobe** • Bricks dried slowly in the sun, but not in direct sunlight, made of clay that has been thoroughly mixed with water, often with straw, grass or other natural fibres added.

**adsorption** • The adhesion, in a thin layer, of liquids to the surface of solids with which they are in contact.

**aerobic** • Living or taking place in the presence of air or free oxygen.

**agency** • Government department, or bilateral, international, non-governmental or similar organization taking primary responsibility for a project.

**aggregate** • Gravel, broken rock or sand that is mixed with cement to make concrete; coarse aggregate particles are normally 6–18 mm in size; sand is known as fine aggregate.

**anaerobic** • Living or taking place in the absence of air or free oxygen.

**aqua-privy** • Latrine in which excreta fall directly through a submerged pipe into a watertight settling chamber below the floor, and from which effluent overflows to a soakaway or drain.

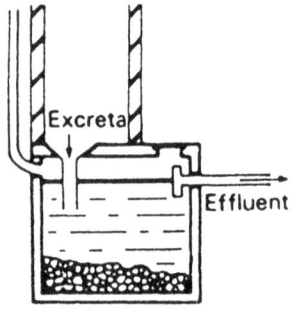

**biochemical oxygen demand** • *See* BOD.

**biodegradable** • Able to be broken down by biological processes through the action of bacteria and other microorganisms.

**biogas** • Mixture of gases, mostly methane and carbon dioxide, produced in anaerobic decomposition of waste materials.

**BOD** • Biochemical oxygen demand: the mass of oxygen consumed by organic matter during aerobic decomposition under standard conditions, usually measured in milligrams per litre during five days; a measure of the concentration of sewage.

**cement mortar** • Mixture of four or fewer parts of sand to one part of cement, with a suitable amount of water.

**cesspit** • A subsurface container for the retention of sewage until it is removed by vacuum tanker or other means.

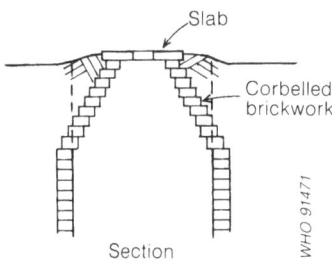

Section

Slab

Corbelled brickwork

WHO 91471

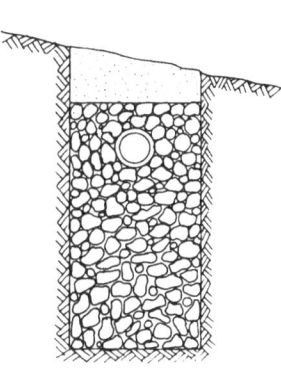

**compost** • Humus produced by composting of organic matter; valued as a fertilizer or soil conditioner.

**composting** • Controlled decomposition of organic solid waste in moist conditions so as to produce humus.

**concrete** • Mixture of cement, sand, aggregate and water which hardens to a stone-like solid.

**corbelling** • Construction in which bricks, blocks or stones are built so that an upper course projects inwards beyond the course below to support a load, such as a manhole cover or squatting slab.

**curing** • Process of keeping concrete or mortar damp for at least the first week after it is cast so that the cement always has enough water to harden.

**decomposition** • Breakdown of organic matter into more stable forms by the action of aerobic or anaerobic microorganisms.

**desludging** • Removing settled solids from pits, vaults, tanks and septic tanks.

**digestion** • Decomposition of organic matter in wet conditions.

**drain** • Pipe or channel for carrying wastewater, effluent, rainwater or surface water.

**drainage field** • Area of land used for infiltration of wastewater into soil.

**drainage trench** • Trench in which a drain is surrounded by stone or other inert material used as a soakaway for liquid dispersion.

**effluent** • Liquid flowing out of a tank or sewage works.

**excreta** • Faeces and urine.

**facultative anaerobe** • Organism that can live in either the presence or absence of air or free oxygen.

**fall** • Slope along a pipe or channel or across a floor, measured as the amount by which one point is lower than a higher point.

**ferrocement** • Cement mortar reinforced by layers of steel mesh.

**flotation** • Process by which solids less dense than water rise to form a scum.

**former (mould)** • Frame, usually wooden, to hold and maintain the shape of concrete while it is setting.

**greywater** • *See* sullage.

**groundwater** • Water beneath the ground surface.

**helminth** • A worm, which may be parasitic or free-living.

**host** • A man or animal in which a parasite lives and from which it obtains food.

**humus** • Decomposed vegetable matter—the end-product of the composting process.

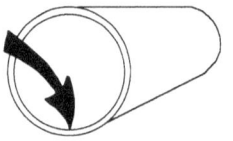
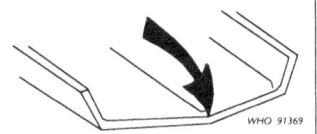

**invert** • Bottom of the inside of a pipe or channel.

**larva** • Worm-like stage of development of insects and helminths, which can move and seek food.

**latrine** • Place or building, not normally within a house or other building, for deposition, retention and sometimes decomposition of excreta.

**mortar** • Mixture of mud, or of lime and/or cement with sand and water, used for joining or for providing a smooth waterproof surface.

**mould** • *See* former.

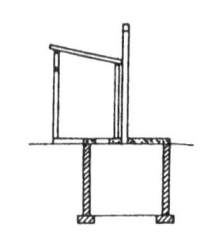

**nightsoil** • Human excreta, with or without anal cleaning material, which are deposited in a bucket or other receptacle for manual removal (often taking place at night).

**offset pit** • Pit that is partially or wholly displaced from its superstructure.

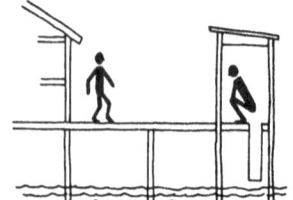

**overhung latrine** • Latrine sited such that excreta falls directly into the sea or other body of water.

**pan** • Basin to receive excreta which are then flushed into an outlet pipe by water poured in or by water delivered around the rim of the pan from a cistern.

**parasite** • Organism that lives in or on another living organism, called the host, from which it obtains its food.

**pathogen** • Organism that causes disease.

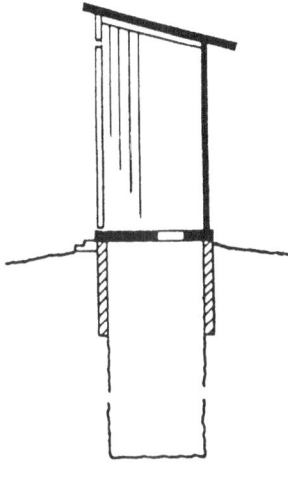

**percolation** • Movement of liquids through soil.

**pit latrine** • Latrine with a pit for accumulation and decomposition of excreta and from which liquid infiltrates into the surrounding soil.

**pollution** • The addition of harmful liquid, solid or gaseous substances to water, soil or air.

**pour-flush latrine** • Latrine where a small quantity of water is poured in to flush excreta through a water seal into a pit.

**programme** • Continuous undertaking for planned objectives with commitment by an institution for long-term support of operation and maintenance; may include a series of projects.

**project** • Planned budgeted event with realizable goals within a specified time period.

**retention time** • Time taken for a volume of liquid to pass through a tank or treatment process, or the time during which a solid or liquid is held in a container.

**sanitation** • The means of collecting and disposing of excreta and community liquid waste in a hygienic way so as not to endanger the health of individuals or the community as a whole.

**screed** • Layer of mortar (usually cement mortar) laid to finish a floor surface.

**scum** • Layer of suspended solids less dense than water and floating on top of liquid waste from which they have separated by flotation.

**sedimentation** • Process by which suspended solids denser than water settle as sludge.

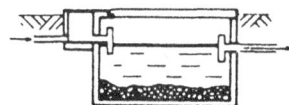

**septic tank** • Watertight chamber for the retention, partial treatment, and discharge for further treatment, of sewage.

**sewage** • Wastewater that usually includes excreta and that is, will be, or has been carried in a sewer.

**sewer** • Pipe or conduit through which sewage is carried.

**sewerage system** • System of interconnected sewers.

**sludge** • Solids that have been separated from liquid waste by sedimentation.

**soakaway** • Soakpit or drainage trench for subsoil dispersion of liquid waste.

**soakpit** • Hole dug in the ground serving as a soakaway.

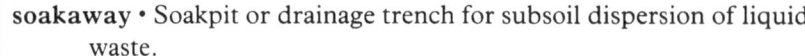

**soffit** • Top of the inner surface of a pipe (also known as "crown") or lower surface of a slab.

**squat hole** • Hole in the floor of a latrine through which excreta fall directly to a pit below.

**sullage** • Wastewater from bathing, laundry, preparation of food, cooking and other personal and domestic activities that does not contain excreta.

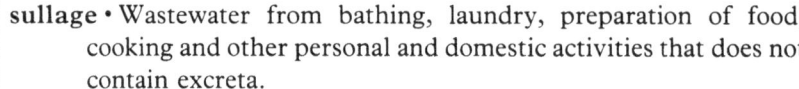

**superstructure** • Screen or building of a latrine above the floor that provides privacy and protection for users.

**surface water** • Water from rain, storms or other precipitation, or street washing lying on or flowing across the surface of the ground.

**toilet** • Place for defecation and urination, which may be the superstructure of a latrine.

**toilet, chemical** • Receptacle used for defecation and urination that contains a strong chemical disinfectant which retards decomposition and reduces smell.

**transpiration** • Loss of moisture by a plant through its leaves.

**trap** • *See* water seal.

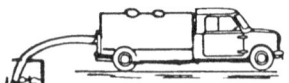

**vacuum tanker** • Lorry-mounted tank into which the contents of septic tanks, aqua-privies, cesspits, vaults or pits are drawn by vacuum pump for transport to a treatment or disposal site.

**vault** • Watertight tank for storage of excreta.

**vector** • Insect or other animal that can transmit infection directly or indirectly from one person to another, or from an infected animal to a person.

**vent pipe** • Pipe provided to facilitate the escape of gases from a latrine or septic tank.

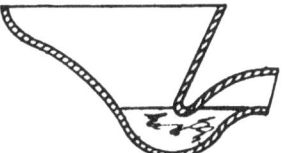

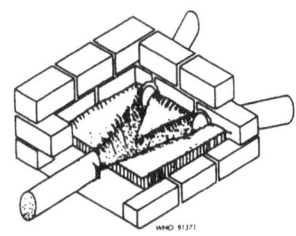

**VIP latrine** • Ventilated improved pit latrine; pit latrine with a screened vent pipe and a partially dark interior to the superstructure.

**wastewater** • Sewage or sullage.

**water closet (WC)** • Pan from which excreta is flushed by water into a drain.

**water seal** • Water held in a U-shaped pipe or hemispherical bowl connecting a pan to a pipe, channel or pit to prevent the escape of gases and insects from the sewer or pit.

**water table** • Surface level of groundwater.

**Y-junction** • Chamber in which liquid may be directed along either of two pipes or channels.

ANNEX 1
# Reuse of excreta

Human excreta should be regarded as a natural resource to be con-
served and reused under careful control rather than being discarded.
Excreta for reuse are derived from:

— nightsoil, including that collected by municipal systems or private
  contractors, and the nightsoil of individual households or groups of
  households and used on their own gardens or farms;
— solids from full pit latrines;
— sludge, scum and liquor from septic tanks, aqua-privies, vaults and
  cesspits; and
— raw and treated sewage and sludge from sewage treatment works
  (which are outside the scope of this book).

Solids from pit latrines are innocuous if the latrines have not been
used for two years or so, as in alternating double pits. Raw excreta from
all other sources are likely to include recently excreted faeces and may
therefore contain active pathogens.

There are three basic methods of using this resource: agriculture,
aquaculture, and biogas production.


## Use in agriculture

Human excreta are a rich source of nitrogen and other nutrients
necessary for plant growth. The most common method of reuse is direct
application to the soil as a fertilizer. Nightsoil contains about 0.6%
nitrogen, 0.2% phosphorus and 0.3% potassium, all of which are
valuable plant nutrients. The humus formed by decomposed faeces also
contains trace elements which reduce the susceptibility of plants to
parasites and diseases. Humus improves the soil structure, enhancing
its water-retaining qualities and encouraging better root structure of
plants. Soil containing humus is less subject to erosion by wind and
water and is easier to cultivate.


### Health risks

For centuries, untreated nightsoil has been widely used as a fertilizer in
east and south Asia, although there is an increasing awareness of the
public health dangers involved. Pathogens of all kinds can remain
viable in the soil and on crops (see Table 2.4, page 14). Death of
pathogens on crops is usually caused by desiccation and direct sunlight,

so pathogens are generally more persistent in humid cloudy climates than in arid areas.

It has been suggested that the use of raw excreta and the effluent from septic tanks is acceptable only if confined to industrial crops and foodstuffs that are cooked before being eaten. However, even with these crops, there is considerable risk of pathogen transmission to agricultural workers, to people involved in transporting crops, and to those processing industrial crops or preparing food for cooking. Therefore such use must be carefully planned with strict surveillance by the health authorities.

The risks arising from pathogen transmission from the use of untreated excreta or sludge on food crops may be greater for populations with high levels of hygiene and health (for example people in towns) than for agricultural workers living in areas where excreta-derived diseases are endemic (Feachem et al., 1983).

### Excreta on paddy fields

Fields with crops standing in water during part or all of the vegetation period are potential transmission sites for schistosomiasis if fresh excreta are used as fertilizer (Cross & Strauss, 1985).

### Fertilization of trees

Treated or untreated sewage is sometimes used to irrigate trees. This practice is most common in arid climates, where trees are watered to control desertification, to provide shade and windbreaks, or to cultivate coconuts and some other food crops. The main health risk is to workers and members of the public who have access to the plantation.

### Excreta on pasture

When excreta are applied to land on which cattle graze there is a danger of the spread of beef tapeworm, whose eggs may survive on soil or pasture for more than six months.

## Composting

Excreta may be treated in various ways to eliminate the possibilities of disease transmission. Apart from storage in double-pit latrines, the most appropriate treatment for on-site sanitation is composting.

Composting consists of the biological breakdown of solid organic matter to produce a humic substance (compost) which is valuable as a fertilizer and soil conditioner. It has been practised by farmers and gardeners throughout the world for many centuries. In China, the practice of composting human wastes with crop residues has enabled the soil to support high population densities without loss of fertility for more than 4000 years (McGarry & Stainforth, 1978).

Nightsoil or sludge may be composted with straw and other vegetable waste, or with mixed refuse from domestic, commercial or institutional premises. The process may be aerobic or anaerobic.

Aerobic bacteria combine some of the carbon in organic matter with oxygen in the air to produce carbon dioxide, releasing energy. Some energy is used by the bacteria to reproduce. The rest is converted to heat, often raising the temperature to more than 70 °C. At high temperatures there is rapid destruction of pathogenic bacteria and protozoa, worm eggs and weed seeds. All faecal microorganisms, including enteric viruses and roundworm eggs, will die if the temperature exceeds 46 °C for one week. Fly eggs, larvae and pupae are also killed at these temperature. No objectionable odour is given off if the material remains aerobic.

In the absence of oxygen, nitrogen in organic matter is converted to acids and then to ammonia; carbon is reduced to methane and sulfur to hydrogen sulfide. There is severe odour nuisance. Complete elimination of pathogens is slow, taking up to twelve months for roundworm eggs, for example.

### Practical composting

The traditional method of composting is to pile vegetable waste with animal manure and nightsoil or sludge on open ground. Aerobic conditions may be maintained by regular turning of the material, which also has the advantage of making the moisture content more uniform throughout the tip. Under aerobic conditions, rapid decomposition of organic matter takes place in the first 2–4 weeks. The process is considerably shorter than under anaerobic conditions. Controlled composting in mechanized composting equipment shortens the process even more.

According to Flintoff (1984) there are five preconditions for successful composting:

— suitability of the wastes;
— marketability of the product;
— support of authorities, particularly those in agriculture;
— a price for the product that is acceptable to farmers; and
— a net cost (i.e., process costs less income from sale) that can be sustained by the operating authority.

#### Pretreatment
In developing countries most domestic refuse is vegetable matter, and there may be little paper, glass or metal. Where these materials are more common, paper can be composted and some glass is acceptable in compost if it is ground up at some stage of the composting process. Metals need to be removed. Textiles, plastics, leather and the like may be removed or they may be shredded and included in the compost. Dust and ash may also be included but, if they form too large a proportion of the refuse, the value of the compost is reduced.

Working over refuse heaps with forks to break down large lumps helps the composting process. Broken-down refuse has a greater surface area for air to enter and for bacteria to attack. It allows less penetration of rain and fly control is easier.

## Control of composting

Too much moisture in a heap of composting material fills the spaces between particles, preventing air from getting in. On the other hand, bacteria do not flourish if the material is too dry. The optimum moisture content is 40–60%. Moisture content can be increased by spraying a compost heap with water, and can be decreased by adding dry straw or sawdust. Frequent turning allows a heap to dry naturally by evaporation.

For optimum value to plants, the ratio of available carbon to nitrogen in compost should be about 20. In the composting process carbon is used by the bacteria, so the best raw material for composting has a higher carbon:nitrogen ratio, say about 30. The carbon:nitrogen ratio of nightsoil is about 6, of fresh vegetable waste around 20, and of dry straw over 100. The ratio of mixed household refuse is often in the range 30–50, but it may be higher if there is a high paper content. The desirable ratio of 30 can sometimes be obtained by judicious mixing of incoming waste, for example by adjusting the proportions of nightsoil or sludge and vegetable waste. It is rarely practical to determine the carbon:nitrogen ratio by chemical analysis; a good operator learns to judge what mix of materials will produce the best compost.

During composting the volume is reduced by 40–80% and the weight by 20–50%.

## Windrows and pits

Unless expensive mechanical plant is used, aerobic composting of municipal refuse is usually carried out in long heaps called windrows. The best height for windrows is about 1.5 m. In heaps more than 1.8 m high, the material at the bottom becomes too compressed; in heaps less than 1 m high, too much of the heat generated by the bacteria is lost.

The width and length of windrows should be planned for the most efficient handling of materials and the best utilization of the area available. The initial width is often 2.5–3.5 m at the bottom. In dry weather the cross-section should be trapezoidal, as shown in Fig. A1.1, but during the rainy season a more rounded shape prevents the material getting too wet.

For composting small quantities (for example, from a single village), refuse should be stored until there is enough to make a pile about 3 m in diameter and 1.5 m deep.

For composting nightsoil, a common method is to place alternate layers of nightsoil (about 50 mm thick) and vegetable waste (about 200 mm thick) in pits or windrows. Fig. A1.2(a) shows how a windrow can be formed to ensure destruction of faecal pathogens by high temperature. Vegetable matter below and at the edges provides some

**Fig. A1.1. A compost windrow**

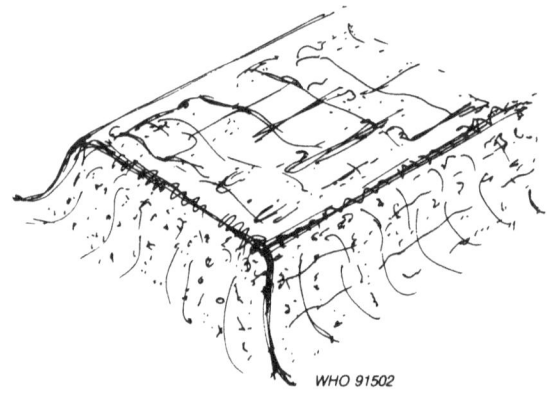

WHO 91502

**Fig. A1.2. Placing nightsoil in a compost windrow**

(a)

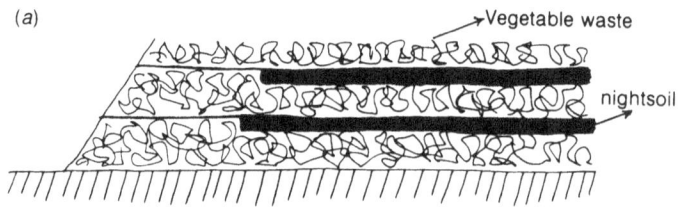

Vegetable waste

nightsoil

(b)

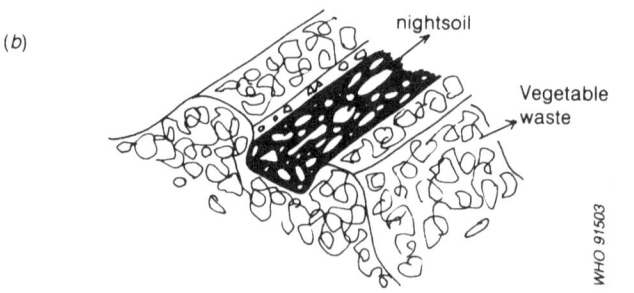

nightsoil

Vegetable waste

WHO 91503

insulation. Fig. A1.2(b) shows an alternative method: after a windrow has been in use for two or three days and the temperature has risen, a trench or pocket is formed in the centre and nightsoil is poured in.

*Temperature, aeration and turning*

Providing that the material being composted remains aerobic the temperature may rise to 45–50 °C during the first 24 hours. A few days later it will reach 60–70 °C, well above the lethal temperature for all pathogenic organisms. Fig. A1.3 shows the variation in temperature during aerobic composting of mixed municipal refuse; the points marked T indicate when the material was turned for aeration.

Various methods of aeration have been tried. For a small refuse heap (as in a village), refuse can be tipped over bamboo or timber poles which are removed when the heap is complete, leaving holes through which air reaches the refuse (see Fig. A1.4). Other approaches, including forced aeration (using compressed air blowers or suction) and use of porous floors, have not been very successful in keeping large masses of material aerated.

**Fig. A1.3. Temperature variation during aerobic decomposition of mixed refuse (T = point at which material was turned for aeration)**

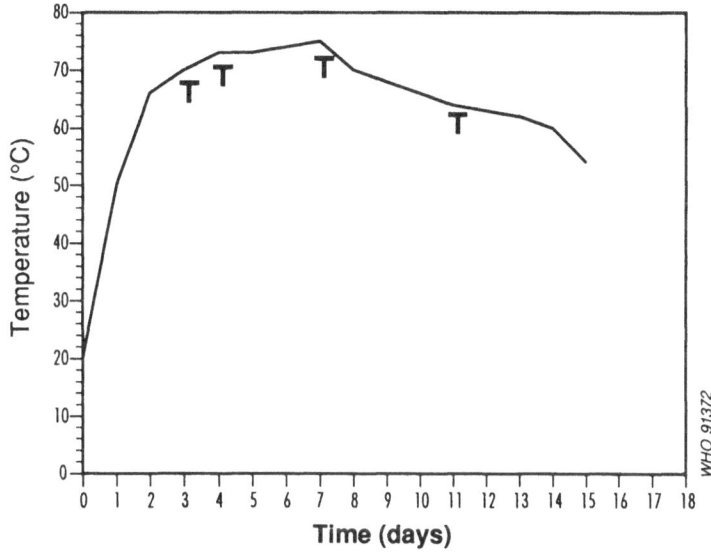

**Fig. A1.4. Aeration of compost by placing around poles**

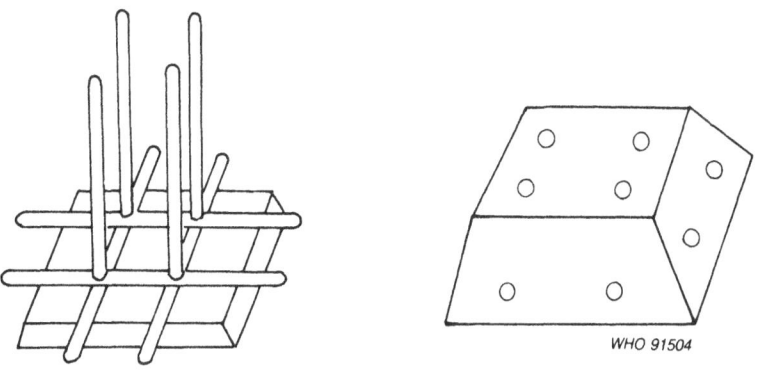

Material in windrows can be turned by labourers using forks or by adapted earth-moving equipment. Turning should keep the heap aerobic. In addition, material at the outside should be moved to the centre, because the outer layers may:

— be too wet because of rain;
— be too dry owing to evaporation (especially on the side facing the wind);
— be unaffected by the temperature rise in the centre of the windrow;
— contain large numbers of flies, fly eggs and larvae.

Some operators turn their windrows every two or three days. However, aerobic conditions can be maintained with less frequent turning after the first week or so. One suggested pattern is to turn the windrow after one day and then on the 3rd, 7th, 14th and 21st days. On the 28th day the material is put into a storage area to await removal.

Generally compost is only required at certain times of the year. If there is only one harvesting and sowing season a year, an area sufficient to store most of the year's production of compost may be required. During storage, compost continues to "mature", but high temperatures cannot be maintained. The time taken for stabilization depends on the initial carbon:nitrogen ratio, the moisture content, maintenance of aerobic conditions and the particle size. Unless precautions are taken, fly breeding may be a problem when compost is stored.

*Condition and quality of compost*
Tests of compost during and after stabilization show whether the process is going well and whether the finished product is suitable for agricultural use. Except in a large mechanical composting plant, the condition of the compost is gauged by simple methods. It is reasonable to assume that pathogenic organisms will be killed if the temperature rises above 65 °C. This can be confirmed by poking an iron bar or wooden stick into the heap and pulling it out after about ten minutes. It should then be too hot to hold. The temperature falls when stabilization is complete. Absence of an unpleasant smell and absence of flies also indicate satisfactory aerobic composting (Flintoff, 1984). An experienced operator can check that all is well from the appearance of the composting material. It should look moist, but not so wet that liquid seeps out. While aerobic stabilization is progressing the appearance will change from day to day. Anaerobic conditions are shown by a pale green, slightly luminous appearance of material inside the heap.

Farmers and market gardeners may want to know the chemical composition of compost derived from nightsoil or sludge. The major plant nutrients (nitrogen, phosphorus pentoxide and potassium oxide) are likely to be about 3% by weight, three times the concentration in compost from municipal refuse.

## Use in aquaculture

The practice of depositing excreta into fish ponds or tanks is common in many Asian countries. In some places, latrines are placed immediately over or alongside ponds; elsewhere nightsoil is tipped from carts, tankers or buckets. Nutrients in excreta result in a rich algal growth, which encourages aerobic conditions and provides food for certain fish.

Carp and tilapia are especially suitable for such ponds, but a variety of fish species may coexist, some feeding on large algae, some on small algae, some on zooplankton; some prefer the bottom layer, some the top. Fish are usually netted for human consumption, but in some places they are dried and ground up for feed for poultry or animals. Ducks may also be kept on the ponds.

There are three health risks associated with fish farming in ponds that receive excreta.

(1) Pathogens may be transmitted on the body surfaces or in the intestines of the fish without causing overt disease in the fish; the pathogens may then be passed to people handling the fish.
(2) Helminths, particularly flukes, may be transmitted to people who eat infected fish that has not been properly cooked.
(3) Helminths with intermediate hosts (such as *Schistosoma* with water snails) may continue their life cycle in ponds.

The WHO publication, *Guidelines for the safe use of wastewater and excreta in agriculture and aquaculture* (Mara & Cairncross, 1989), gives further useful information.

## Biogas production

The search for alternative sources of energy has led to widespread use of organic waste to produce a combustible fuel which can be used for domestic cooking. Basically, a biogas plant consists of a chamber in which excreta are fermented, producing gas which contains about 60% methane. The biogas is collected at the top of the chamber, from which a pipe leads to domestic appliances or to flexible storage containers.

A few biogas plants operate entirely on human excreta. For example, in Patna, India a 24-seat pour-flush latrine serves several thousand people and generates sufficient energy to light a 4-km length of road. However, most plants, of which there are more than 7 million in China (Li, 1984), are dependent on animal excreta with which human excreta are processed. A medium-sized buffalo or cow provides about twenty times as much gas as a person. The minimum feed is that from one cow and a family of people, although it is more usual to add excreta from at least four cows. In China it is customary to produce biogas from the excreta of pigs.

## Construction

Although there are many variations, the most common types of domestic plant have a floating or fixed dome under which the gas collects. The floating dome type, shown in Fig. A1.5, is widely used in India. In China, masonry or concrete fixed domes are usual, as shown in Fig. A1.6. They are generally cheaper than those with a floating roof. The daily gas output is approximately equal to one-third the volume of the digester.

**Fig. A1.5. Biogas plant with floating dome**

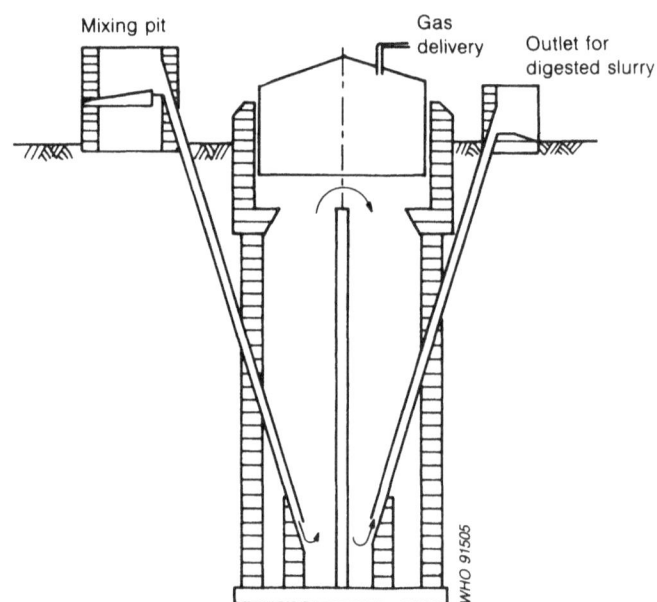

**Fig. A1.6. Biogas plant with fixed dome**

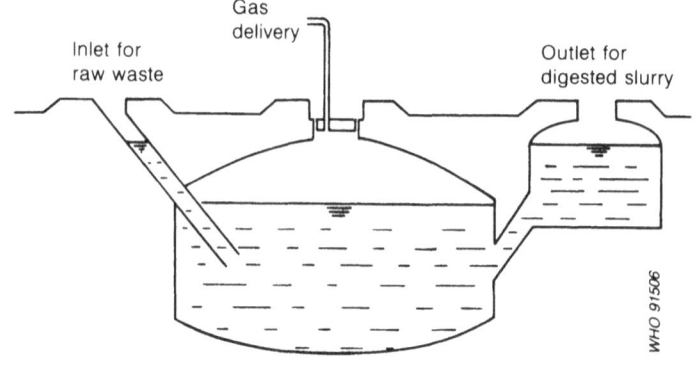

## Operation

Excreta are often mixed with straw or other vegetable waste, such as that used for animal bedding, and equal quantities of water added to make a slurry. This is fed to the inlet side of the chamber. Effluent slurry is removed after a retention time of 30–50 days. Biogas production is greater at higher temperatures. At 30 °C the rate of generation of gas is about twice that at 25 °C, and little gas is produced if the temperature is below 15 °C.

The effluent slurry is usually dried in the open and used as a fertilizer. On a dry solids basis, the nitrogen content is greater than in untreated excreta because of the loss of carbon in the gas. The nutrients in effluent slurry, whether dried or applied directly to land, are more readily taken up by plants.

## Health risks

Retention of excreta in biogas tanks results in the death of many pathogens, including *Schistosoma* eggs. A few hookworm eggs survive, and there is high survival of roundworm eggs.

## References

CROSS, P. & STRAUSS, M. (1985) *Health aspects of nightsoil and sludge use in agriculture and aquaculture.* Dübendorf, International Reference Centre for Waste Disposal (IRCWD Report No. 04/85).

FEACHEM, R. G. ET AL. (1983) *Sanitation and disease: health aspects of excreta and wastewater management.* Chichester, Wiley.

FLINTOFF, F. (1984) *Management of solid wastes in developing countries*, 2nd ed. New Delhi, WHO Regional Office for South-East Asia (South-East Asia Series No. 1).

MCGARRY, M. G. & STAINFORTH, J. (1978) *Compost, fertilizer, and biogas production from human and animal wastes in the People's Republic of China.* Ottawa, International Development Research Centre.

MARA, D. & CAIRNCROSS, S. (1989) *Guidelines for the safe use of wastewater and excreta in agriculture and aquaculture.* Geneva, World Health Organization.

# ANNEX 2
# Sullage

Sullage is domestic wastewater other than that which comes from the toilet. It results from food preparation, personal washing, and washing of cooking and eating utensils and clothes. It is also called greywater (to distinguish it from blackwater which describes wastes containing human excreta).

There are few published studies of the characteristics of sullage in developing countries. Research in the United States of America has shown that sullage has a lower nitrate content than toilet wastes, and a more soluble and more biodegradable organic content (Laak, 1974). The suspended solids load in sullage is lower than in wastes from toilets, but it contains more grease and is generally at a higher temperature. Kitchen wastes have a higher suspended solids content, a higher biochemical oxygen demand, and a higher nitrate concentration than other sullage.

The volume and characteristics of the sullage produced by one community may be very different from those of another. A family served only by a remote standpipe or handpump may discard less than 10 litres of sullage per person each day, whereas members of a household with numerous plumbing fixtures may discard 200 litres each or more per day. In some countries, rivers or lakes are used for personal hygiene and for washing clothes and utensils, so that the volumes of wastewater leaving the house are low. Table A2.1 shows the water consumption measured in rural households, demonstrating a wide range of consumption rates.

The nature of the sullage is markedly influenced by factors such as diet, methods of washing clothes and utensils, habits of personal hygiene, and the existence of bathrooms and other facilities.

There are several reasons for keeping sullage separate from excreta. First, there may be a system for on-site disposal of excreta that cannot accept large volumes of water. Alternatively, the sullage may be transported away from the site by a small-diameter pipe that could not handle faeces. A third reason might be to reduce the hydraulic loading on a septic tank by diverting the sullage away from it (Bradley, 1983).

Sullage is discharged or disposed of in a number of ways. Often it is simply tipped on to the ground in the yard or outside the property where it evaporates or percolates into the soil. It may be used to irrigate a vegetable or flower garden. It may find its way by natural or designed routes into open or subsurface storm drains. Soakpits or drainage fields may be built to disperse the sullage. In some cases the greywater from a

**Table A2.1. Water consumption (litres per person per day) in some rural areas in four developing countries**

| Water use | Lesotho[a] | Uganda[b] | | Pakistan Punjab[c] | Mozambique[d] |
|---|---|---|---|---|---|
| | | Lango | Kigezi | | |
| Drinking and cooking | 8.0 | 5.8 | 6.4 | 5.7 | 2.3 |
| Other domestic use | 10.0 | 11.9 | 1.6 | 24.0 | 10.0 |
| Total | 18 | 18 | 8 | 30 | 12 |

[a] Feachem et al., 1978
[b] White et al., 1972
[c] Ahmed et al., 1975
[d] Cairncross, S., personal communication.

number of properties is collected, screened and treated in ponds before it is discharged or reused.

## Health implications of sullage management

In general, the health hazards posed by sullage are not as serious as those associated with either wastewater containing excreta or septic tank effluent. Counts of faecal indicator bacteria have been reported to be significantly lower in sullage than in septic tank effluent (Bradley, 1983), but the washing of babies' clothes and nappies (diapers) is likely to increase the count substantially. Some data suggest that bacteria grow well in sullage (Hypes, 1974).

A substantial danger from pathogens is posed by careless tipping of greywater on the ground. If one particular area is always used, its continual moistness will favour the survival of helminths, such as hookworm, and the breeding of flies and mosquitos. In addition, such an area is more likely to be regarded as a waste dump and so be used for defecation, and this practice will increase the number of parasites. Faeces are not easily seen when the ground is muddy.

The main hazard to public health is posed by mosquitos, especially *Culex quinquefasciatus*, which breed in polluted pond water and may spread bancroftian filariasis. Ponding of sullage is caused by excessive discharge on to the ground, by blockage of surface drains, or by unsatisfactory construction or maintenance of open channels to carry the sullage.

Pollution of groundwater by sullage may be of less concern than the pollution threat from other wastewater, because the bacterial and nitrate contents are relatively low.

It is often thought that the provision of a more abundant supply of water to a community will necessarily bring about an improvement in health. However, if the greater availability of water causes the creation of pools of stagnant sullage (because sullage disposal has not been carefully considered), then the improved water supply could have a negative effect on the health of the community, largely as a result of the increase in the mosquito population. The disposal of sullage is a particular problem at communal water points. Often, large volumes of wastewater are generated and, if provision is not made for its proper disposal, a significant health hazard may develop.

## Disposal of sullage

Pouring sullage on to the ground can be an acceptable means of disposal provided that the soil is not continually moist. This means that the soil must have sufficient permeability and be of adequate area to allow the sullage to percolate away. This method of disposal can be put to good effect by using the sullage to irrigate vegetable gardens, but vegetables that will be eaten raw should not be watered with sullage because of the danger of disease transmission.

Infiltration through field drains or soakpits, as used for the disposal of septic tank effluent, is suitable for sullage. The size of soakpits and trenches may be designed using the long-term infiltration rates shown in Table 5.4. Examples 8.6 and 8.7 in Chapter 8 explain the design of infiltration systems.

Sullage often finds its way, by accident or design, into open drains. Such drains can be a satisfactory method of conducting the sullage to a body of receiving water provided that there is no ponding of sullage in the drains. Pools encourage mosquito breeding, and children often play in them. Ponding is likely to occur where the terrain is flat and the drain slope small, where the drains are rough and unlined so that water collects in depressions, where refuse is deposited in the drains, and where drains are filled in to allow vehicles or pedestrians to cross.

Storm drains that are also used for transporting sullage should have a compound cross-section as shown in Fig. A2.1. This is because the flow of stormwater in the rainy season can be hundreds of times larger than the flow of sullage alone. A simple cross-section designed only for stormwater would conduct the sullage away at a very low velocity, leaving the solids suspended in the sullage in the bottom of the drain. The circular channel in the invert of a compound cross-section allows small flows to move at a higher velocity. Drain-cleaning tools should be adapted to fit the small central channel.

### Fig. A2.1. Cross-section of a compound storm drain

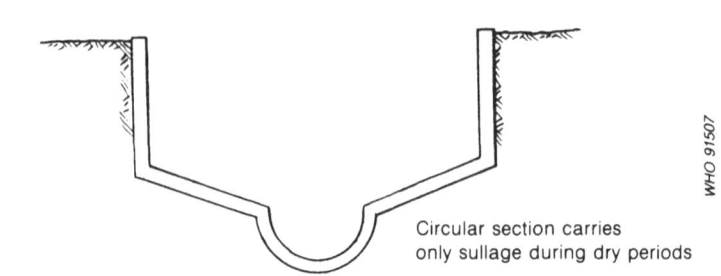

Circular section carries
only sullage during dry periods

WHO 91507

Keeping drains free of refuse is not easy. Unfortunately it is commonly believed that a drain is an appropriate place for depositing solid waste, especially where there is no adequate refuse collection service. Refuse in drains quickly becomes malodorous as it decomposes and is attractive to flies as a site for egg-laying. Removal of such material from the drains is not a popular task. The problem of solid waste in open drains calls for a three-pronged attack:

— the provision of a satisfactory refuse collection service to provide an alternative outlet;
— public education, especially on the need to keep the drains clear; and
— vigilance on the part of municipal labourers to remove blockages wherever they occur.

In one city in Brazil, each householder was made responsible for keeping the length of drain outside his or her property clean; grilles were fitted at points in the drains in line with the dividing walls between the properties so that no refuse could be carried on to a downstream neighbour's section, and any flooding occurred in the area where the refuse was deposited (Cairncross, personal communication). Grilles of this type have also been used in other countries, installed by the municipal authorities or by residents to prevent refuse entering the sections of drain for which they are responsible.

Covering the drains may appear to be a solution, but if refuse is deposited in the drains through gaps or by lifting cover slabs, the resulting blockages and ponding are much harder to detect and clear.

Small-bore sewers can be used to convey sullage. Diameters and slopes can be less than those recommended for sewage containing excreta because the solids load is less. Where sand is used for scouring cooking pots it may be necessary to install traps to collect this grit before it goes into the sewer. However, attention must be given to ensuring that these traps are emptied periodically—the mere provision of them without adequate maintenance is not enough. There may also be a risk of grease deposits building up in the pipes. Grease traps can be used to separate grease from the rest of the wastewater, but they are only effective if the accumulated grease is removed at regular intervals. Generally, grease traps are fitted at garages, restaurants and other commercial premises where large quantities of oil or grease are discharged in the wastewater (Fig. A2.2).

Sullage can be treated on site to make it more acceptable for final disposal or reuse. Septic tanks can be used; they are effective in removing grease and solids, and do not require frequent desludging (Brandes, 1978). Intermittent sand filters are effective in reducing biochemical oxygen demand and nitrate levels, but Boyle et al. (1982) found they had little effect on the numbers of faecal indicator bacteria.

The selection of the most appropriate sullage disposal system depends on many factors, such as rainfall, soil structure, topography, housing density, water consumption, latrine type, and a variety of social and economic factors. For example, where there is sufficient yard area,

**Fig. A2.2. Cross-section of a grease trap**

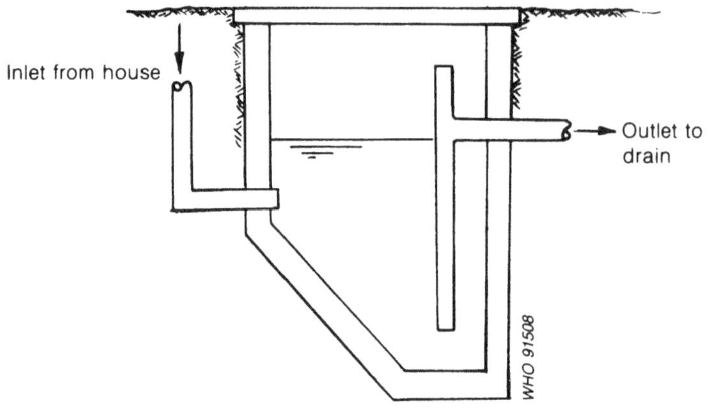

the soil is permeable, the rainfall is such that ponding never occurs, and sullage is produced in small quantities, it may be quite satisfactory to pour the sullage directly on to the soil. Where the subsoil permeability, housing density and income permit, a soakpit is recommended. Alternatively the sullage could be disposed of in a pit latrine, where one exists. Where there is sufficient slope for surface drains, and the ability to keep them free of debris has been demonstrated, disposal to these drains might be acceptable as an interim measure, provided the drainage system has an appropriate discharge point. Small-scale pilot studies are often valuable for assessing the suitability of the various alternatives before implementation on a large scale.

The main problems posed by sullage are socioeconomic rather than technical in origin. Most disposal systems only function correctly if operated and maintained in a proper fashion. This is particularly evident in surface drainage systems where the agencies responsible for maintenance are often under-funded and thus unable to carry out their duties adequately. In such circumstances, the maintenance must be taken over by the community—but the community must first be convinced that clean drains are necessary for good health.

# References

AHMED, K. ET AL. (1975) *Rural water consumption survey*. Lahore, Institute of Public Health Engineering and Research (Report No. 026-12-74).

BOYLE, W. C. ET AL. (1982) Treatment of residential greywater with intermittent sand filtration. In: Eikum, A.S. & Seabloom, R.W., ed., *Alternative wastewater treatment*. Dordrecht, Reidel, pp. 277–300.

BRADLEY, R. M. (1983) The choice between septic tanks and sewers in tropical developing countries. *The public health engineer*, 11 (1):20–28

BRANDES, M. (1978) Characteristics of effluents from grey and black water septic tanks. *Journal of the Water Pollution Control Federation*, 50 (11): 2547–2559.

FEACHEM, R. G. ET AL. (1978) *Water, health and development: an interdisciplinary evaluation.* London, Tri-Med Books.

HYPES, W. D. (1974) Characteristics of typical household greywater. In: Winneberger, J. H. T., ed., *Manual of greywater treatment practices*, Michigan, Ann Arbor Science, pp. 79–88.

LAAK, R. (1974) Relative pollution strength of undiluted waste materials discharged in households and the dilution waters used for each. In: Winneberger, J. H. T., ed., *Manual of greywater treatment practices*, Michigan, Ann Arbor Science, pp. 68–78.

WHITE, G. F. ET AL. (1972) *Drawers of water.* Chicago, Chicago University Press.

# Reviewers

Dr N. O. Akmanoglu, WHO Centre for Environmental Health Activities (CEHA), Amman, Jordan

Professor S. J. Arceivala, Associated Industrial Consultants, Bombay, India

Dr S. Cairncross, London School of Hygiene and Tropical Medicine, London, England

Mr J. O. Espinoza, WHO Regional Office for Europe, Copenhagen, Denmark

Mr K. Gibbs, United Nations Children's Fund, Quetta, Pakistan

Dr I. Hespanhol, World Health Organization, Geneva, Switzerland

Professor K. O. Iwugo, University of Lagos, Lagos, Nigeria

Mr K. Khosh-Chashm, WHO Regional Office for the Eastern Mediterranean, Alexandria, Egypt

Dr H. Kitawaki, World Health Organization, Geneva, Switzerland

Mr J. N. Lanoix, Consultant Sanitary Engineer, Sarasota, FL, USA

Dr G. B. Liu, WHO Regional Office for the Western Pacific, Manila, Philippines

Dr P. Morgan, Blair Research Laboratory, Harare, Zimbabwe

Mr A. F. Munoz, Pan American Center for Sanitary Engineering and Environmental Science (CEPIS), Lima, Peru

Mr C. Rietveld, World Bank, Washington, DC, USA

Mr A. K. Roy, Consultant Sanitary Engineer, New Delhi, India

Mr L. Roy, Consultant Sanitary Engineer, Neuilly-sur-Seine, France

Mr R. Schertenleib, International Reference Centre for Waste Disposal, Dübendorf, Switzerland

Dr G. S. Sinnatamby, Senior Sanitary Engineer, United Nations Centre for Human Settlements, Nairobi, Kenya

Mr M. Strauss, International Reference Centre for Waste Disposal, Dübendorf, Switzerland

Mr M. S. Suleiman, World Health Organization, Geneva, Switzerland

Mr H. Suphi, WHO Regional Office for South-East Asia, New Delhi, India

Dr S. Unakul, WHO Western Pacific Regional Centre for the Promotion of Environmental Planning and Applied Studies, (PEPAS), Kuala Lumpur, Malaysia

Mr J. M. G. Van Damme, International Reference Centre for Community Water Supply and Sanitation, The Hague, Netherlands

Dr D. B. Warner, World Health Organization, Geneva, Switzerland

# Index

www.ingramcontent.com/pod-product-compliance
Lightning Source LLC
Chambersburg PA
CBHW080126150626
46550CB00017B/2690